blue
rider
press

EVERY DAY I FIGHT

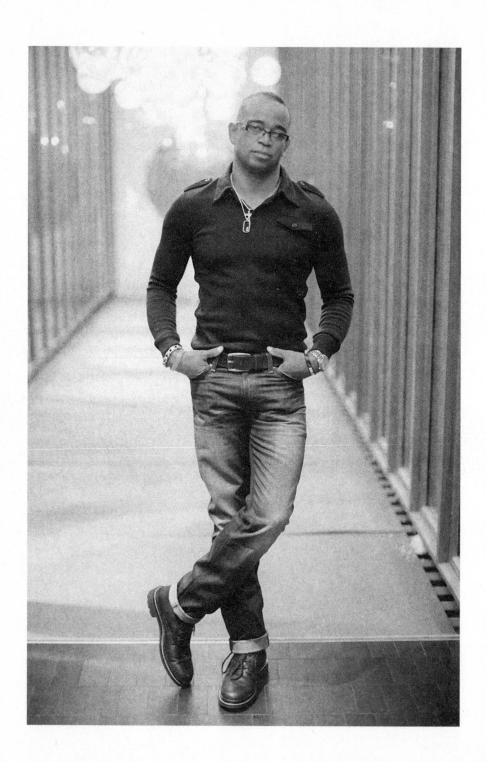

EVERY DAY I FIGHT

STUART SCOTT

with Larry Platt

BLUE RIDER PRESS

New York

blue
rider
press

Blue Rider Press, a Penguin Random House imprint
375 Hudson Street
New York, New York 10014

USA · Canada · UK · Ireland · Australia
New Zealand · India · South Africa · China

penguin.com
A Penguin Random House Company

Library of Congress Cataloging-in-Publication Data

Scott, Stuart, 1965–2015.
Every day I fight / Stuart Scott, Larry Platt.
p.   cm.
ISBN 978-0-399-17406-3
1. Scott, Stuart, 1965–2015.   2. Sportscasters—United States—Biography.
3. Cancer—Patients—United States—Biography.   I. Platt, Larry.   II. Title.
GV742.42.S35A3   2015   2015002612
070.4'49796092—dc23
[B]

Printed in the United States of America
1   3   5   7   9   10   8   6   4   2

BOOK DESIGN BY CLAIRE NAYLON VACCARO

About the front jacket photograph: Stuart Scott sat for Dear World, a portrait project
founded by Robert X. Fogarty. In his distinct message-on-skin style, Fogarty asks
each subject to share a message about something or to someone they love.

For Taelor and Sydni

Yes, Stuart Scott was as cool as the other side of the pillow. But he was so much more than the hippest sports journalist ever. It wasn't just his unique catchphrases that set him apart. Stu was also one of the most authentic people I have ever been blessed to know. Simply put, he was the real deal on and off camera. We met in 1993. I had been at ESPN for a few years by then, and Stu was hired to be an anchor for the launch of ESPN2. Our cool factor went off the charts with Stu roaming the halls and performing "Rapper's Delight" on karaoke nights. He brought a spirit and a style that had never been seen, never been felt before, at ESPN.

Stu and I hit it off right away and discovered we had a lot in common. We both were from the South, were college hoops fanatics, and were the youngest of four children in our families. It was apparent that Stu came from a good, loving, and supportive family. Soon he started a family of his own. Taelor and Sydni were his world. Oh, how he loved being their dad. He proudly showed us their pictures as they grew into beautiful, talented young women. He'd whip out his phone and show us the latest video of them performing. Taelor playing the guitar, Sydni singing. Nothing, and I mean nothing, made Stu happier or brought him more pure joy.

Later Stu and I shared something else in common. Cancer. But that never was the focus of our conversations. We didn't feel the need to talk about it. There's an unspoken language and understanding between those facing cancer. You focus on the fight, not the fright. Every day he fought for his girls . . . before and after he became ill. I'll never forget when his cancer returned for a third time. I went with him to the gym to watch him train. He had taken up martial arts and cross-training workouts. In the midst of grueling chemotherapy treatments, it was his way to treat his body as well as his spirit. The punches and kicks he threw were physical as well as symbolic. It was Stu's way of continuing to battle, to literally kick cancer's you-know-what!

After the workout, he began bragging about Taelor and Sydni. Then he told me: "I want to be here because I don't want some other dude walking my daughters down the aisle at their weddings." Those girls gave Stu purpose in his life and his fight.

Though the outcome was not what we wanted, not what we prayed for, Stu's fight was every bit as valiant and meaningful. Like many, I remain in awe of how he stared cancer smack-dab in the face. Sitting in the audience at the ESPYS, I marveled at how he found the strength to get out of his hospital bed and take that stage. It was incredibly fitting that he received the Jimmy V Award for Perseverance. Jim Valvano and Stuart Scott were cut from the same cloth. Two dynamic men who embraced life and changed lives. That night at the ESPYS, Stu must have been the bus driver, cuz he was takin' us to school. He delivered an invaluable lesson for the ages: "When you die, it does not mean that you lose to cancer. You beat cancer by how you live, why you live, and the manner in which you live." His words were as raw, honest, and powerful as the man himself.

Stu's unshakable courage was inspirational. Cancer never defined him; it's not his life's story but rather a chapter in his life's story. You'll see in these beautifully written pages that he set a stellar example for all of us in so many aspects of life. Stu said when you're too tired to fight, rest and let someone else fight for you. My dear friend, you can rest now, and we will continue to fight for you.

ROBIN ROBERTS

EVERY DAY I FIGHT

WHY I FIGHT

My phone was blowing up. The text messages were coming nonstop, and, with each one, I was feeling more and more like an imposter. There were hundreds of them, almost all using words like "courageous," "brave," "inspirational."

Only I felt like none of those things. No, the only thing I felt, the only thing I've ever felt since the day in 2007 I learned that what I thought was appendicitis was actually a rare form of cancer, was . . . fear. To readers of that morning's *New York Times*, I may have seemed courageous. But trust me: I ain't courageous. I just don't want to die.

The article, on this March day in 2014, was headlined "A Story of Perseverance: ESPN Anchor's Private Battle with Cancer Becomes a Public One" and it had all the background. It had the three surgeries that had removed my appendix, large intestine, some lymph nodes, other organs; the fifty-eight infusions of chemotherapy I'd undergone to that point; the Wound VAC that drained the foot-long scar that ran from chest to belly button and that had taken two months to heal after a ten-hour surgery in the fall of 2013. And it had me wearing a black "Everyday I Fight" T-shirt at the mixed martial arts studio near my Connecticut home, where I go straight from chemotherapy to jab and hook and kick until I collapse, drained.

But that's not courage. That's survival. When cancer storms into your life, you have a choice: fight, or curl up and just be a cancer patient. That doesn't mean I don't have my moments. There are times when I say to myself, *It's too much, I don't have the energy for this fight.* There are times I bawl my eyes out and tell my girlfriend, Kristin, who has slept on a cot by my bedside throughout countless hospital stays, "I'm scared, I'm really scared." I come from jockdom; what guy likes being that vulnerable? I have many such moments, but they're not the *last* moment I have. And they're not my most enduring moments.

Because having cancer, it turns out, is more complicated than you'd think. Like any great opponent, cancer is in your face. It practices the art of intimidation. It gets inside your head and messes with your thinking. It takes its toll on you physically, but the real burden is mental. I've told my doctors I don't want to know my prognosis: "I'm not interested in hearing how long *you* think I *might* have." That would be just another thing to be frightened of and obsess over.

But let's keep this real. I'm forty-nine. There's a good chance I'm going to die a helluva lot earlier than I ever wanted to. There's a good chance I'm going to die soon. And I know it. I know it every moment of every day. And that reality is never *not* with me.

So this book is a chronicle of my fight against cancer, but it's even more than that. It's really a memoir of a life well fought; in sports, the media, or the cancer ward, the one true thing I've learned is that life is hard but that there is redemption in the struggle.

Cancer is just the latest, and most terrifying, fight. Though I hate this most unwanted of companions, I respect it for its power—and there are even times when I'm grateful for what it's given me. Don't get me wrong: From day one, I was committed to beating it. But along the way, I've learned how paradoxical the relationship between patient and disease really is; cancer turns the old cliché on its head. It can kill you *and* make you stronger, all at the same time.

That's why words like "brave" don't really apply when confronting cancer. When you first hear that you have it—a doctor prefaced breaking the news to me by saying, "Things just got more complicated"—you say to yourself: *I'm going to die.* And, in my case, the very next thought was even more of a sledgehammer: *I won't be here for my two daughters.* After a while, once the sting subsides, you ask yourself: *How do I fight cancer?*

Here's what I knew about cancer: You get it, you die. But I'd always been a competitive sonofabitch. I turned down a couple of football scholarships out of high school to attend my dream school, the University of North Carolina, where I was friendly with Michael Jordan before he was the greatest who ever lived; I planned on being a walk-on wide receiver there, but an eye disease, keratoconus, ended my collegiate career before it began. As a sports broadcaster debuting on ESPN in the early nineties, I brought the in-your-face attitude of the music I came up on—hip-hop—to *SportsCenter.* That wasn't a planned thing; it was just who I was. Yeah, I'm young, I'm African-American, and I'm telling you about this game like I'm talking trash with my boys back home: *"Man, Mike about to put it on these boys! Mike about to mess them up!"* Even my most famous catchphrase—*Boo-yah!*—was all about capturing those adrenaline-fueled moments of intimidation in sports.

Yet behind the on-air bravado was a craftsman; I actually kept a running chart of how many statistics colleagues like Keith Olbermann, Dan Patrick, and Chris "Boomer" Berman used in their broadcasts because I was determined to lead the nation in giving the audience cold, hard facts behind the loudness. You could hate me for my style, but my substance was going to be beyond reproach.

On the football field or the TV set, the only way I knew how to succeed was to push myself, to be stronger than my opponent, to work harder. But now there I was, forty-two years old, and the opponent before me was a freakin' assassin. How do you work harder than cancer? I didn't know. But when I want to work hard, I go to the gym. After my first four-hour chemo treatment, I was hooked up to a two-day chemo drip in a little bag that attached to a port in my stomach—and thirty minutes later, I was in the gym. On the elliptical machine, I looked down and noticed the name of the medicine dripping into my body: It was called fluorouracil, or 5-FU for short.

I smiled, said a little prayer, and then stuck that pack into the pocket of my gym shorts and said to myself: *FU, cancer.* The athlete in me realized: This thing growing inside me was trying to kick my ass. Well, I've gotta hit first and kick *its* ass. So I attacked the elliptical and made a promise to myself: From then on, I'd be working out within thirty minutes of each chemo treatment. Later, I'd skip the gym—there were too many inquiries about my health; they were well-meaning, but we members of the alternative universe that is CancerWorld chuckle at the overly earnest, stage-whispered "how you feeling" queries meant to convey deep concern—and instead I started doing P90X or mixed martial arts in the living room of my house. From day one, working out was my own private "FU" to cancer.

Because cancer is trying to rob the most precious thing in the world to me: time with my daughters, Sydni, fifteen, and Taelor, nineteen. They're why I say "FU" to cancer every day. When I have those moments—when I say to myself, *This is too hard, I'm too tired to go on*—I remind myself that cancer forced me to reconsider my life's goal and that I haven't reached it yet: I want to walk Taelor and Sydni down the aisle. I don't want them with an uncle or some father figure; that's my place.

I hate that a group of abnormal cells inside my body has such control over my life. At the same time, I can't deny that cancer has actually given me something. Because it gives every moment meaning. Because I'm on a time clock and I don't know what that time clock says. And no moments are deeper than those with my knuckleheaded daughters, for whom I fight every day.

A FEW WEEKS AGO, Sydni came home—I share custody with my ex-wife—and asked if her girlfriends could come over and get ready with her for that night's dance. And, of course, could I drive them to it?

Hell, yes. "Do you want me to get some chips?" I called to her.

"Sure, Dad," she said. "Get some chips." I could almost hear the eye roll through her closed bedroom door. Sydni is beautiful and talented—she's the soloist in her school choir—but she's at that age where anything Dad does, by virtue of him having done it, is uncool.

On our way to the dance, the classic old-school tune "Cameosis" by Cameo came on. I reached for the volume and cranked it up, bellowing, "Now, this is when music was music!" and started singing along:

> *When you hear a group that moves you*
> *And feel it in your feet*
> *You ask yourself, hold on a minute*
> *What group now can this be.*

The girls were all laughing, but Sydni wasn't having it: "All right, Dad, whatever," she said, insisting on a newer sound track. Kendrick Lamar came on, and now the girls were the ones singing, Sydni most of all, all of them smiling—they were showing the old man something.

And I just looked at them through that rearview mirror and thought: *This is so cool. I'll never do something more important than this. Taking my daughter and her friends to a dance.*

This is what cancer does. It makes you look fresh at small moments and see them—really see them—as if for the first time.

Pre-cancer, the ride to the dance would have been merely fun, and then I wouldn't have thought about it again. But it wouldn't have hit deep. It wouldn't have seared into my mind's eye the image of Sydni's smiling, singing face.

During Super Bowl week last year, I met Taelor for lunch in New York City. She was between classes at Barnard College. We sat there, my firstborn and I, as she chatted away: about an assignment for sociology, her roommate, a boy who might possibly like her. My phone was vibrating, again and again. The old me would have answered. There's always time for my girls, after all, right? Not the cancer me. *Let it go, man,* the cancer me said. Nothing's more important than being with this person who, together with Sydni, changed my life more than anyone. Later, Kristin would say: "I called you today," and I'd reply: "I was with Taelor." 'Nuff said.

I'm not trying to "Kumbaya" you. My daughters are *teenagers,* man. Sydni is in perpetual eye-roll mode and Taelor is a typical college student; she'll call for advice or to ask for money or to share a joke—only, of course, not as often as her needy Dad wishes she would. Teenage girls are a whole 'nother thing. They get angry with me, annoyed, embarrassed. Friends tell me they'll come around. Teenage girls always come around to their dad eventually.

But that well-meaning advice strikes to the heart of my fear. I don't have "eventually." The truth is, I'm not as afraid of dying as I am of not being here for my daughters' aha moment. I'm on the clock and I want to be here when they get it—when they get what I got about my dad: that all the stuff he did that ticked me off? He did that *for* me.

Ray Scott was a federal postal inspector—the dude carried a gun and cuffs; I'd grow muscles when the neighborhood kids would see him. He promised his four kids that he'd pay our college tuition if we maintained a 2.0 grade point average. After my sophomore year, I was skating along with a 2.7. Dad said he was restructuring our deal—he'd only pay if I kept a 3.0 or better. "That's crap," I said. That wasn't the deal. It wasn't fair—a common refrain from my teenagers today.

But then something happened: In the fall of my junior year, I was heavily involved with my fraternity, I played club football, *and* I posted a 3.2 GPA. The next semester, I upped that to 3.6. The following one, 3.4. I remained pissed until years later, when it dawned on me: Dad *knew* I was better than a 2.7 student. And he knew I needed to be pushed. Funny, isn't it, how much smarter our dads are when *we* get older?

That was my aha moment about my dad. Will Sydni and Taelor have theirs about me in time? Maybe that's selfish of me to wonder. Maybe their aha moment about me is for them—not me. But I can't help myself. I want them to realize that everything I do, I do with their best interests at heart—and I want that to happen while I'm still around for them to talk to me about it, like I did with my dad.

This is what cancer does. It makes everything profound. It makes everything urgent.

A COUPLE OF YEARS AGO, during a game of the NBA Finals, a couple of security guards were escorting Sydni, Taelor, and me through the concourse; we were on our way to see the family of a friend who was an NBA executive. Because I'm on TV, I tend to get recognized when I'm out, but this was a sports-centric crowd, so I was being swarmed. As fans saw me, they started to call to me. Some asked for autographs. One guy planted himself in front of me.

"Sorry, man," I said, "can't—in a hurry," as security helped us sidestep him.

"You're an asshole!" he called out.

I laughed. Taelor was shocked: "Dad, that guy called you an asshole!" she exclaimed. "I mean, you *can* be an asshole, but he doesn't know that!"

I cracked up. But back at *SportsCenter*, the anecdote prompted a bull session hypothetical. A bunch of middle-aged sportscasters started to wonder: What would it take for each of us to throw down?

"Man, someone calling me a name or cross-eyed, that's funny," I said. "That ain't worth stepping outside."

Now, I know how to fight. I train. I know how to punch, how to kick. But you're not going to call me a name and get me to fight.

Then the question came: What would you do if someone called one of your *daughters* a name? I paused. "I'd put him down," I said.

That might sound like a contradiction, but it's actually very calculated. I want my girls to see me walk away if someone calls me a name. But I also want them to know that I won't let anybody mess with them. I want them to know I'll protect them. Maybe I'm wrong. But I feel this overwhelming need to show them how much I'm willing to fight for them.

And that's what I'm doing every day against cancer: fighting for them. This book is about my fight against cancer, yes, but it's also about why I fight, whom I'm fighting for, and how I find the energy to stay in the ring.

It's also about the central paradox of that fight: You hate this thing inside you. You want to rid your body of it. At the same time, you're aware of what it's done to you: how it gives you an urgency to live—really live—every day; how it makes you see the profound in the everyday; how it teaches patience and humility. The contradiction is as top-of-mind as the fact of the cancer itself: Cancer can kill you, but it can also make you the man you always wanted to be.

CHAPTER ONE

FATHER'S DAY

t's funny what people think. If you look at Twitter, it won't take you long to find some outraged accusations of bias against ESPN. A good amount of them have been directed at me. We're not impartial journalists, the conspiracy theorists suggest; we pick and choose certain leagues, teams, and players to support. I've been accused of kissing up to LeBron, Tiger, or, back in the day, Michael. As a network, we've been said to favor the SEC, act as a publicity arm for Tim Tebow, and bow down before King James.

It always makes me laugh, because it's just so naïve. We're a ratings-driven business, so why wouldn't we have devoted ample coverage to, say, Tebow when his story was top-of-mind throughout the nation? That's called journalism, folks. My colleagues and I—we're journalists. We cover what *you're* interested in.

Now, I also happen to be a sports fan. And I'm very transparent about the fact that I root like hell for my North Carolina Tar Heels, because I bleed Tar Heel blue. But do I pull for LeBron? Hundreds, maybe even thousands, of Twitter comments suggest that I do—in pretty graphic terms. I like LeBron as a person and I respect him as an athlete, but the fact is, James's teams the past few years have been the pulse of the NBA—and *that's* why he has received so much attention from us.

During the 2013 NBA Finals, I took some heat on Twitter after the San Antonio Spurs beat the Heat by 36 points in Game Three. I tweeted: "San Antonio fans in downtown . . . Ur team won game 3 . . . they DID NOT win the title. Stop honking horns, driving slow & yelling out cars. Go Home!!"

Man, Twitter blew up. You would have thought I'd nominated LeBron for sainthood. The irony is that those in the Twitterverse who were accusing me of bias then were kind of right a year later. When I decided to write this book, I committed to keeping it real with you. So it's confession time: During the 2014 NBA Finals, I violated the journalist's code of objectivity. I *was* rooting for someone to win. And I was pulling harder for that outcome than I ever have.

But it *wasn't* the Heat I was cheering for with all my might. After the Spurs took Game One, I wanted them to win the title. And I wanted it desperately. By Father's Day, with the Spurs leading James's Heat 3 games to 1, I had never wanted a team to wrap up an NBA title more than the San Antonio Spurs. But that had little to do with being a sports fan. And even less to do with basketball.

"WATCH HOW THE BALL doesn't stick," I said.

"What do you mean, 'doesn't stick'?" Sydni asked.

"It never stops in one place; they use the whole court," I said. It was that pivotal Game Five, and we were courtside. I was showing Sydni what I love about the way Gregg Popovich's San Antonio Spurs play the game. "It's art, watching these guys play basketball."

Sydni isn't a die-hard basketball fan, and she tends to keep her emotions inside—unlike her old man. Oh, she was interested, but she wasn't consumed by the experience. Again: unlike her old man. To be sitting there with my baby girl, on Father's Day, watching a championship happen . . . and to host the postgame trophy presentation with Sydni standing just a couple of feet from the podium, it was suddenly too much: *This*, I said to myself, *this is what I live for.*

I found myself choking up. I was moved by a confluence of factors: Father's Day, Sydni's smiling presence . . . and the fact that I was about to show off for my daughter. She was about to see her dad do what he does better than anyone on the planet.

Go ahead and alert the ego police: I know I sound less than humble. A lot of times, on the *SportsCenter* set, I blurt out: "*I love my job!*" Often, I look at my colleagues and say, "Can you believe we get paid to do this?" I love it, and I love being among the best in the world at what I do. I wasn't always good at it. But I've worked at it. And I'm damn proud about how I do it.

Now, as Sydni and Taelor will be only too happy to tell you, that doesn't mean there ain't a host of things their dad sucks at, but if there's one thing I know I can do, it's the live interview. I'm maniacal about it; watch a game with me in my living room and you'll hear me shouting "*Dumb question!*" at the TV when a microphone is put in an athlete's face just after he or she has come off the field of play. It's one thing ESPN does better than most networks, because we think deeply about the kinds of questions that can elicit memorable and insightful postgame moments.

Everyone tends to make the same mistakes. They ask questions that lead directly to yes or no answers. They rush to fill the silence when an interview subject is thinking. *"Wait! Just wait!"* I'll scream at my TV. They'll ask a question and then breathlessly answer it: "Coach, why did you double-team LeBron—were you trying to make his teammates beat you?" They'll ask generic questions: "Coach, tell us about the third quarter, when you blew the game open." I'm always waiting to hear the coach say in response: "Well, why don't you *ask* me a question about the third quarter?"

Focusing on specific moments leads to memorable answers. I hate when an athlete is asked, "You just won a championship—how does it feel?" I fantasize about the response: "I just won a championship—how the hell you *think* it feels?" There are ways to ask the "how do you feel" question without literally asking it. When LeBron won his first title, I said to him: "LeBron, when the clock hit triple zeroes, what was the first thing that ran through your mind?"

He didn't miss a beat. "About damn time," he said—instantly an iconic response.

Early on at ESPN, I was interviewing Tiger Woods. I forget what I asked him, but it made him think—so much so that he was silent. *Uh-oh*, I remember thinking, *this is uncomfortable 'cause he's not answering.* I was so afraid of the silence that I panicked and gave him an out by blurting out another question. We had a consultant at ESPN who showed me the tape and asked, "Why'd you ask that second question?"

"Well, he wasn't answering," I said.

He smiled knowingly. "So wait," he said. "Just wait."

I've never forgotten that. If you hate sports interview clichés

like I do, then the silence that comes while a subject thought-
fully constructs a real response is not something to be afraid
of—it's actually a good thing. It means you're going to get something real in return. And this doesn't just apply to sports interviews. Ever seen *All the President's Men*? Now, I'm not comparing
myself to journalists who took down a president, but in that
film, *Washington Post* reporters Bob Woodward and Carl Bern-
stein, played by Robert Redford and Dustin Hoffman, unearth
information from sources by letting their subjects fill the silence.
Most people want to be understood; the journalist's job is to ask
questions that make subjects think—and then to get the hell out
of the way.

So I spent Father's Day preparing for that night's trophy presentation, in the event that the Spurs prevailed—as I hoped they
would. In the hotel room or at lunch with Sydni, I was constantly scrawling questions on the back of an envelope that I
hoped would make Tim Duncan and his teammates resist the
usual platitudes and instead say something real and memorable.
Like the athletes who would take the court that night, I spent the
day aware of my increased heartbeat and fluttering stomach, familiar sensations that told me I was getting ready for the big
stage. I like being nervous. When Taelor competed in dance and
Sydni in soccer, I would tell them, "Nerves are good." What are
nerves, after all? They're just energy.

So, as we got to the arena and ran through rehearsal a few
hours before tip-off, I'd pause every once in a while to focus on
the nerves: I'd identify them as energy, focus on that dropping
sensation in my gut, and tell myself to take that energy and use
it. That's what I'd tell Sydni before a big game or Taelor before

a dance recital: Take the nerves, manipulate them into energy, and make them work for you.

In my inside jacket pocket, I kept the envelope on which I'd scrawled some questions. I spent the day obsessively tweaking, retweaking, and memorizing them. When the final buzzer sounded, and the Spurs had routed the favored Heat, the fans started pressing onto the court; I told Sydni to stay right by the podium. And then I got up on that stage and knocked that mutha outta the park. Keeping in mind that good questions are also short questions, I asked unlikely series MVP Kawhi Leonard, "If I would have told you before this NBA Finals started that you would be the MVP, you would have said what?"

"I would have said, 'You're crazy,'" said Leonard, an unassuming guy off the court who turns into a warrior on it. And then I weaved in some stats and a smooth segue. Saying good-bye to Kawhi, I said, "Kawhi Leonard, MVP, the youngest Finals MVP since 1999, when a guy named Tim Duncan won the MVP. That's what we call a segue—Timmy, where are you?"

Later, off the podium, I asked Duncan, "At what point in the game did you allow yourself to realize, 'We got this'?," and he thought for a moment before responding: "You know, it took a while. When that last sub came in, I got subbed out and I got to the sideline and that's when I let myself feel it."

While the Spurs doused one another in champagne, I said good night to America and climbed down from the podium to my daughter. Like the athletes on the stage, I had that familiar adrenaline high. There's no rush like the one that comes from a momentous live TV shot, especially when you know 18 million people are watching. I was high from a job well done, yes, but also because of what it all *meant*. The moment had special significance to me. A year ago, when the Heat outlasted the Spurs in Game Seven, I hadn't been on that podium.

The day after Father's Day 2013, I was having serious blockage issues. Before my entry into CancerWorld, I never would have thought that going to the bathroom would become such an integral part of my life. But my whole schedule revolves around planning to or needing to get to a bathroom—a logistical challenge when you host a nightly live TV show. By then, I'd gone through two major surgeries in which many of my organs had been resected—the large intestine, the small intestine, part of the colon. As a result, I can no longer digest food normally. I can eat only the blandest of foods, and even then, whenever I eat, you can hear the constant rumblings of my stomach. But by Game Five, I knew my distress was more than mere indigestion. I was blocked, I was in pain, and I knew what it meant: I'd either developed scar tissue from those past surgeries, or yet another tumor was announcing itself.

It killed me to leave, but I had no choice. Instead of the party-like atmosphere of South Beach for Game Six, I was headed for the all-too-familiar accommodations of New York–Presbyterian Hospital. In the fall, I'd have a ten-hour operation there to remove more cancerous masses. For now, my terrific team of doctors treated my symptoms for five days. From my hospital bed I watched our sideline reporter, Doris Burke, host the trophy presentation on the podium after Game Seven. Doris is a consummate pro and she did a great job. But I've got to tell you, watching it, I wasn't a happy camper. The NBA Finals trophy presentation is a big deal and it only happens once a year. And I love doing it. And here I was, watching it from a damned hospital bed. "That's *my* job," I said to myself. I was ticked off. Cancer was keeping me from doing my job. Cancer was keeping me from doing the thing I love. Freakin' cancer. I clenched my fists and vowed I'd be back on that podium in a year.

And now here I was, just off it, putting my hands on each of Sydni's shoulders, smiling ear to ear. "Guess what?" I said. "Now I get to fly home—with you!" More time with my daughter— the real reason I was pulling so hard for the Spurs.

That, and the fact that this meant I could finally start a new clinical trial at the Johns Hopkins Hospital in Baltimore. I'd been trying to start this trial—an experimental type of chemo— for over a month. But before each session, you have to take a scan, and something called the bilirubin and ALT have to be at certain levels in your blood work in order to proceed. I was going to start the trial two days before the 2014 Finals began, but my blood work didn't qualify. So during the Finals, I got my blood checked in San Antonio—and my levels were good. The trial runs every two weeks; looking at the schedule, that would have been the day after Game Six in Miami. So, had the Heat won Game Five, I would have had to part company with Sydni and fly back to Miami from San Antonio for Game Six, after which I'd work until one in the morning, then charter a plane to Baltimore so I could be at Hopkins by the eight a.m. clinical trial start time . . . all to sit in a soft recliner for hours while poison gets pumped into my body. And then, in the event the Heat forced a Game Seven, I'd fly to San Antonio for that.

Phew. I would have done it. Happily. But the Spurs came

through, and now you know why I was pulling for them. Take that, Twitter nitwits.

FRIENDS AND FAMILY MEAN WELL; they really do. They frown when they hear of my schedule—like the jet-setting I would have had to do had the Spurs not closed out the series—or when they see me on *SportsCenter* night after night. *Shouldn't you just be resting?* they might wonder. Some might sheepishly inquire, "Have you thought about taking some time off?"

Uh, no. Man, from the minute I was diagnosed in 2007, I didn't want to be the cancer patient who is sitting at home, unable to work. This is what I do. It's who I am. If I'm too weak to work, I'm admitting that I'm too weak to live. I'd be miserable. If I didn't travel, if I didn't work, if I didn't exhaust myself doing mixed martial arts or P90X in my living room, if Kristin and I didn't don boxing gloves and spar after poison has been shot into my body, I guarantee you I would have succumbed to cancer years ago.

After my diagnosis, I looked up appendiceal cancer once on the Internet, and I vowed to never research it again. The statistics flashed before me: how rare it is, affecting between 600 and 1,000 people per year, and how deadly—the five-year survival rates are not favorable. Why would I seek out such information? It would only scare me more. And that's when I decided that, yes, I'm going to trust my doctors and my medicine, but that's not how you beat cancer. You beat cancer by continuing to live. By refusing to be *just* a cancer patient.

For the past seven years, I've very consciously tried to model perseverance for Taelor and Sydni. If they can see me working hard, if they can see me not quitting, that's something they can take with them for the rest of their lives. As I've said, it's not courageous—it's born of necessity. If you want to stay here, you have no choice but to fight.

But I honestly believe that my lifelong apprenticeship in sports helped prepare me for this mother of all challenges. You know the story of Louis Zamperini, right?—the "unbroken" Olympic runner and World War II veteran whose story of survival, resilience, and redemption was chronicled in a bestselling book and brought to the big screen by Angelina Jolie. Before his death last year at ninety-seven, Zamperini said that his athletic training helped him overcome the beatings and torture he endured at the hands of the Japanese during his years as a prisoner of war. "You have to learn self-discipline if you are going to succeed as an athlete," Zamperini said when asked to reflect on how he got through those years. "For another thing, you have to have confidence in yourself and believe that no matter what you're faced with, you can deal with it—that you just can't give up. And then there's the aspect of staying in shape. And humor helped a lot, even in the gravest times."

Hear, hear, Louis. I learned early on from sports that resilience makes all the difference in life. I knew it when one of my earliest idols, Muhammad Ali, got dropped by Smokin' Joe Frazier in the fifteenth round of their first epic fight. It was a punch that would have kept anyone else flat on the canvas. But back up came Ali, struggling to his feet. He might have had more triumphant moments, but no truly greater one, because nothing ever so valiantly displayed such a pure fighting spirit.

But Jim Valvano's great ESPYs speech in 1993 really made me realize that there are lessons for the ages in our moments of struggle and challenge. I'm a Carolina guy, a Tar Heel through and through. After college, I covered North Carolina State for WRAL-TV in Raleigh, North Carolina, when Coach V was going through a recruiting scandal at State. One of my first big one-on-one interviews came during that time, when Coach V sat down with me at his house. We sat out back and his wife brought us lemonade, and when the camera switched off, we talked about life. It dawned on me that he'd had rivalries with Duke and my beloved UNC, but I couldn't think of any Dukie or any Tar Heel who didn't genuinely like Jimmy Valvano.

So maybe I was predisposed to be moved by his speech because of my affection for him, but I don't think that was it. I think it was his words, it was his defiance, it was his attitude despite the odds. Think about those words: the simplest yet most poignant seven words ever uttered in any speech anywhere: *Don't give up, don't ever give up.*

I was just starting at ESPN at the time and had just gotten married. My wife, Kim, a flight attendant, and I would soon be starting a family. I remember hearing Valvano's words and thinking: *That's the key to life.* It was like someone grabbing you by the collar and saying, "Hey. Don't. Give. Up. Not now. Not ever."

Say what you will about Lance Armstrong—I think he did whatever everybody else in his sport was doing, and that it shouldn't tarnish his accomplishments on a bike—but what is undeniable is that here was a world-class athlete who got cancer in his brain *and* in his nutsack. And he basically said, "Screw that. I'm getting off this table." I dig that. I played sports all my life and I dig that attitude. *Okay, you're hurting? Get up anyway.*

I dig it when I see it at any level. A couple of years ago, Sydni was in a big soccer match and an opposing player took her out with a cheap shot. She landed on her shoulder, which had already been injured the year before, and wasn't moving. They have this dumbass rule in her soccer league that if your kid gets hurt, you can't run onto the field. Well, I didn't ask. I ran full speed to her while her coach called out, "Stuart, you can't be here."

Screw that noise. That's my baby girl in a heap. When I got to her, I bent down and said, "Babe, I'm here." And you know what she said? Crying and in pain, she blurted out: "Dad, get off the field!" Later in the game, she lumbered back onto the field. She wasn't running fast, but she got up, dusted herself off, and came back for more.

That's my girl, I thought. I love that moment.

Remember Sam Mills? Talk about resilience. Sam was a 5'9" linebacker who made a career of proving his doubters wrong. Along with Reggie White, he was arguably the best defensive player in the USFL, and he went on to become a five-time NFL Pro Bowler with the New Orleans Saints and Carolina Panthers, the last time in 1996 at age thirty-six. As inspirational as his football achievements were, it's what happened after his playing days that made Sam one of my role models. We got friendly when he was a defensive coach for the Panthers in the early 2000s. He was diagnosed with intestinal cancer in 2003 and was told he had only a couple of months to live.

What did Sam do? He did what Sam did. He fought like hell. He'd go from chemo straight to the gym—for a hellacious workout. He continued to coach and was an inspirational force behind the Panthers' run to Super Bowl XXXVIII. He lived two more years, but more important, he *truly* lived, getting the most out of each day. He did it his way. We were kindred spirits.

These are the reasons, culled from a life in sports, that I knew early on I couldn't be just a cancer patient who takes his medicine, goes to chemo, and lies around feeling sorry for himself. I haven't allowed myself a single *Why me?* moment. Because, if I start asking *Why me?* as it relates to cancer, I'd have to start asking *Why me?* as it relates to all of my good fortune: Why was I able to do this job I love? Why was I blessed with Sydni and Taelor and such a great family? Once you start questioning the bad stuff that comes your way, you have to start questioning the good—and I wouldn't trade the good for anything.

Now, that doesn't mean there aren't days when I lie around doing nothing. I'm always on the go; after all, at work and as a parent, my life is full of deadlines. But on the days when Sydni stays at her mom's, I may work out and then spend the rest of the day on the floor in my living room, watching *24* or *Homeland*. Fighting cancer takes energy—and there are moments that require its conservation. Kristin will say, "What do you want to do today?" And I'll reply: "Nothing." She knows that means it's recharging time.

Cancer is complicated, man. Every day, I'm on edge, waiting for the next shoe to drop. Any little pain, and I'm like, *Oh my God, is that cancer? Has it spread? Is it growing?* It's an every-day thing. That's why I seek out, and love, my moments of peace:

Eating cereal on my couch late at night, my all-time favorite movie will come on and I'll sit back and watch that most unlikely philosopher prince, Rocky Balboa, exhibit the character traits I still aspire to. Sitting on a beach, listening to the waves, just *being*. Driving my black E350 Benz on a warm, late summer evening, blaring some old-school LL Cool J, the sound track to *West Side Story*, or Mumford & Sons. Being on a plane . . . and hearing a baby crying. That's the sound of *life*, man. Moms: Stop apologizing for your kid crying—he or she has a right to be there. I love to revel in the beauty of a baby's cry.

All these things make me stop and say: *I love this.* Though football is my first love as a sport—to this day, I've never grown tired of throwing a football around—since getting cancer, golf has become my sanctuary. As much as I love working out and mixed martial arts, golf makes me feel like less of a weak-ass cancer patient than anything else. On the links, the fresh air filling my lungs, I feel free and at peace. On the golf course, I think of cancer less than at any other time, and I'm more defiant in its face. Yes, defiant, because I'm sure cancer doesn't want me feeling so good.

That's why, when I made it to Baltimore for the first clinical trial session after the Spurs spanked the Heat last spring, I brought along a 7-iron and a couple of balls. After the poison entered my vein and started coursing its way through my body, I stepped outside the hospital and dropped my ball on the side of a busy road. On the other side were woods. If you were some dude who happened to be driving through Baltimore that day, you might have seen some crazy-ass golfer hitting a couple of drives over traffic into the woods. And if you could read lips, you might have seen that he said, after his last swing, "*FU, cancer.*"

CHAPTER TWO

TAKING HITS

was nine years old when I took my first hit. And I loved it.

It was on the football field. I was number 34 on the Mount Tabor Tiny Falcons in Winston-Salem, North Carolina, where I grew up. I played outside linebacker and wide receiver.

A week before our first game, I was trying to tackle Larry Dulin; he wasn't a big kid, but he was bigger than me, and he'd had some momentum going when we collided head-on. Both of us went down; I sprained my wrist on the play—it would be the first time I'd wear an Ace bandage, which I thought was the coolest thing in the world. Though I felt the hit all over my body, I remember springing right back up and thinking, *Wow. That's cool.* I immediately liked the contact, the physicality. I liked the anticipation of collision followed by the sensation of it, and I was never afraid of getting hurt. I sensed that the body at top speed was naturally braced for impact. Now I know that my instinct was dead-on: In football, as in life, the hits you *don't* see coming are the ones that do the most damage.

Really, I'd fallen in love with football before I even played a down. Before we moved to Winston-Salem for my dad's job, we were in Chicago, where I was born. One day, when I was four years old, my dad returned from a business trip with a present for me and my older brother, Stephen: an orange football with white stripes on either end. The first memory of my life is of Stephen and me tossing the football to each other on our front lawn and asking Dad, "Can you come out and play with us?"

He always would. Stephen and I were recently talking about our dad, and we both had the same memory of the only time he said no, he couldn't play with us. Ten minutes after he'd refused us, the front door opened. Here came Dad, hands outstretched, calling for a pass.

I realize now how monumental that was. How many kids can say their dad was always there for them? I'm not sure Sydni and Taelor can say that, despite how much I try. Yes, I fell in love with football on the field. But I think I was conditioned to love football at four years old because my dad gave me one and threw it around with me. And my dad was Superman.

OUR HOUSE ON BENBOW Street, about twenty minutes from downtown Winston-Salem, was a 1,200-square-foot ranch. I shared a room with Stephen, two years my senior, while my older sisters, Susan and Synthia, bunked together. It was close quarters, but I never felt cramped or crowded. All I felt was the thrill of all the possibilities to come, and that's a testament to our folks, Ray and Jackie Scott.

We moved to our all-white neighborhood in January 1972 from the all-black South Side of Chicago. I was six; Susan, the oldest sibling, was thirteen. I know now that our lifestyle might have been characterized as lower middle class, but back then? Man, in Chi-town, we'd been in an apartment and then a town house. Here we had a house with a lawn that led to some woods—perfect for exploring. And we never wanted for anything.

Just a year before our arrival, the Winston-Salem/Forsyth County Schools were desegregated. That made us pioneers. Every team we played for, every classroom we entered, we seemed to break our town's color barrier. But here's the thing: We were aware of it, but ol' Ray and Jackie never made a big deal of it. At school, we never entirely fit in, not with the white kids, and—having come from the North—not always with the few other black kids. At home, we embraced the fact that we were different.

We didn't watch *American Bandstand*. We watched *Soul Train*, "the hippest trip in America." For us, Don Cornelius was the slick embodiment of cool. We listened to gospel, Nat King Cole, and Ray Charles. And tons of musical sound tracks. On Saturdays, we'd all have to clean the house while the songs of *West Side Story*, *The Wiz*, and *Godspell* filled the air.

As a parent today, I tell Sydni and Taelor all the time that I want to be the best dad in the world. My mom and dad never told me they wanted to be the best. They just were. For example, back then, there was no such thing as a black angel for the top of your Christmas tree. Well, that didn't stop Mom. She would take shoe polish and make our angel look like us. Same with greeting cards; she'd take a brown pen to them. She didn't say, "Look, they're black, just like you." She'd just do it. It was subtle, but it told us to be proud of who we were.

Because we didn't always get that message outside the home. When we moved to Winston-Salem, I was in the first grade. Our first week of school, my dad and Rascal, our German shepherd, would meet Stephen and me halfway on our mile-long walk back home. On the first day that we made that trek by ourselves, we passed a house with a statue on its front lawn of a small black figure holding a lantern. A lawn jockey, I'd come to learn. On the porch stood a group of white kids, staring us down.

"*Nigger! Nigger!*" they shouted at us, through bared teeth.

Stephen and I knew the word and felt the hate. But we also knew another word.

"*Honky! Honky!*" we called back, with as much venom in return as we could come up with.

The white boys looked quizzically at one another. Then, as if on cue, they turned to us and started shouting this latest epithet back at us: "*Honky! Honky!*" It was as if they figured, *Well, whatever this word is, it must be degrading—so let's call them that!* Stephen and I burst into laughter as we continued on our way, leaving them totally perplexed.

Here's the thing, though: I remember this incident, sure, but I also remember that, at the time, I didn't feel hurt or victimized. I credit my parents for that. Something had been instilled in me that wasn't going to let the irrational anger of strangers make me doubt my own identity. Even in first grade, I wasn't going to be a victim.

A little over a year ago, I got some heat for something I tweeted: "True racism is group w majority/economic/political power discriminating against others . . . Blacks/Hispanics can be ANGRY/RUDE but not 'Racist.'" Man, you can guess how that went over. But I stand by it. Racism is the institutional manifestation of prejudice. Black people can be prejudiced and ignorant, yes, but since blacks by and large don't control our institutions, they don't have the power to act on those impulses, to *subjugate* others. This is something I learned forty years ago in Winston-Salem. I don't care if someone—white or black—doesn't like me because of what I look like. If they can *act* on that dislike in a way that harms me, then we've got a problem.

Growing up, we heard as much ignorance from blacks as from whites. My siblings and I didn't just look different from the white kids; we also didn't sound like the black kids. We were in the South with flat, Midwestern accents—and we came from a household that heavily valued education. As a result, we'd often hear from our black classmates, "You talk like a white boy." All four of us got that all the time. Later, I'd come to realize how hard it is for people who are poor and whose parents aren't educated to value education; then, it hurt, because who we were seemed so often to be in question. It was like we were constantly being asked *Whose side are you on?* in some race-based game we didn't fully understand.

Another time, in fifth grade, a group of popular sixth-grade white boys started letting me hang with them. "You're a cool guy," one boy said. "We're not going to call you Stuart anymore; we're going to give you a nickname."

Cool, I thought: acceptance.

"We're going to call you Sambo," he said. Now it was my turn to not know the meaning of a racial slur. That night at dinner I told my parents I'd made some new friends and they had even given me a nickname: Sambo. At the drop of the word, my folks looked at each other. *Uh-oh,* I thought. *Something's up.* They looked angry, but I could tell they weren't angry with me. They explained to me that Sambo was an offensive term and that these boys weren't my friends. "It's like they're calling you *nigger*," I was told.

Again, I wasn't bothered by it. But what must have this been like for Ray and Jackie Scott? Years later, I got a taste. When Taelor was five we were at one of her dance recitals. After the recital, the parents left the girls to let them play together in the school's basement. As I was heading up the stairs, I heard a bloodcurdling, screeching cry; as a parent, you recognize your kid's cry. I about-faced and jumped down a flight of stairs, sprinting to my little girl, who was crying and gasping for breath. She was the only black child in the troupe and one of the other little girls had just told her, "We don't want to play with you because you're black."

The other little girl's mother seemed mortified and apologized profusely, swearing her daughter hadn't learned that attitude at home. But I admit I wasn't hearing it. I remember wishing that little girl's dad was there so I could beat him down. Even now, fourteen years later, I feel rage. Because I couldn't protect my five-year-old little girl from experiencing her first taste of bigotry. I tear up now, just thinking about it. Is that what Ray and Jackie felt? That sense of crippling parental helplessness?

Kids are resilient, though. Like Taelor when she was five, I eventually shrugged off the incidents in my youth practically as they happened. The day after I told my parents of my new "nickname," Ray Scott, handcuffs hanging off his belt loop and gun holstered, made an appearance at school. I don't know who he talked to or what he said, but thereafter those boys didn't say anything to me ever again. Which was okay—the moment I'd learned they were playing me, I'd already moved on. In fact, I sensed a little bit of fear coming from them after my dad made that visit. You don't mess around with Superman.

RAY SCOTT IS SLOWED by Parkinson's now, but he was and remains the man. My whole life, he radiated dignity, respect, character, and honesty. Pops was a serious man. To this day, I've never heard him raise his voice, but he was very firm. When he told you to do something, you did it. Growing up, I had friends who would sneak out of their houses late at night to party with their friends. I've talked to my siblings about it—it never crossed our minds to do something like that, because of Dad.

First, we were not totally convinced he would not take our lives. That's only a slight overstatement. Remember, we're talking about a law enforcement official. He talked in a level voice that, accompanied by his direct stare, intimidated. He didn't even know he did this, but his eyes would flicker when he got worked up. He'd bat his eyelashes and that, juxtaposed against the eerily calm tone, hinted at just enough menace beneath the surface that we wouldn't think of defying him. He wouldn't yell, but you only had to be spanked by Ray Scott once to want to stay on his good side.

Looking back on it, Dad's spankings hurt, but disappointing him hurt more. I was crushed to think my Superman was disappointed in me. I mean, this dude was a federal law enforcement officer—how cool is that? Postal inspectors work with FBI and ATF agents. When I was in high school, he spent six months undercover in New Orleans, posing as a postal worker named Franklin Baxter in a post office that had been corrupted by a drug cartel. At the end of his assignment, he had to arrest all these people he had worked with and, in some cases, befriended.

That's the literal definition of integrity. I watched him closely, stirred by his eloquent example. He'd get up every morning and run seven miles, come back and meticulously enter his time and route in a log he kept on his desk. He was seen as the neighborhood problem-solver. When our neighbors found that their son had run into trouble with drugs and petty crime, it was Dad they turned to for help.

Everyone seemed to trust him, which I took pride in. When he'd show up at school, with those handcuffs on his belt and that gun holstered, I'd be all like, "Check out my dad," trying to get my friends to see that my dad had theirs beat in the badass department.

Once, when I was seventeen, I was driving the family car—a 1979 Pontiac Bonneville. I had my gangsta lean on (like the soul man said: "*diamond in the back/sunroof top . . .*"), and I might have been testing the speed limit just a bit when the flashing blues and reds came up on me from behind. Now, I was a black man in the South, and my folks had had "the talk" with me. No, not the one about the birds and bees. This one is about the black man and the police. It's a conversation that takes place in black households throughout the country, where driving while black is always a very real threat. My folks taught us what you do when you get pulled over: Flick on that dome light. Hands on the steering wheel. When the officer approaches, you do as Richard Pryor counseled—you announce your intentions: "Officer, I'm about to reach into the glove compartment for the registration."

But there was a problem. As I started to open it, I saw my

dad's gun. I shut the glove box, and my hands went back on the steering wheel.

"Officer," I said. "My father is Ray Scott, federal postal inspector."

"You're Ray's boy?" he said.

Phew. "Yessir, and I want you to know that this is his car and his gun is in the glove compartment."

He let me off with a warning and a message to say hello to my dad. Driving home, I felt nothing but a sense of pride that my dad commanded that kind of respect.

I'm convinced that my dad, in everything he did, was a better man than I'll ever be. And it wasn't just my dad: A whole generation of guys—Tom Brokaw called them the Greatest Generation—were all about what a man should be. We're losing them at a rate of 1,500 per day now. I love seeing them, walking among us in their ratty cardigans and Members Only jackets, because they're a reminder of what they did—and how their Boomer and Gen-X sons and daughters have come up short.

They were the good guys who saved Democracy and then rebuilt the countries they had defeated. They created the greatest economy in history, based on values like shared sacrifice and responsibility. They made successes of themselves, but refused to shut the door behind them. Like Ray Scott, they saw everything in terms of right and wrong.

From Jackie Scott—nicknamed Jackie Baby as a kid—I got my sensitive side. When she was young, she was painfully shy. But she started to find her voice with my father. She spent decades as a public school kindergarten teacher's aide, during which time she earned a reputation as one of those people who likes everybody and whom everybody likes. My mom never had an enemy. How many of us can say that? Dad could be stern, but Mom was a sweet woman who cared—and worried!—about everyone.

They've always had an amazing relationship. They were good, churchgoing people who were aware of the Biblical admonition that "the head of a wife is her husband." Dad used to shake his head at that one. "The best relationships are relationships where the woman lets the man live with the illusion that he runs the household," he'd say.

"Your mom is smarter than me," he'd tell us. "She's better than me." He thought she'd saved him. He was a quiet, tough kid from the Chicago streets when they first met. She smoothed him out, helped open his heart. He, in turn, gave her confidence.

They got married in 1958, and the passion never seemed to wane. Marvin Gaye's song "Sexual Healing" came out when I was in high school, and whenever it would come on, Dad would grab Mom in the kitchen and start dancing. "Hey, I'm right here, okay?" I'd bark, and they'd laugh.

Mom had a way of making everything special, in a very understated way. When I was thirteen, I idolized Stephen. But Stephen, at fifteen, didn't always want to be saddled with his younger brother. One weekend, he and his buddy Sam from across the street were going to Atlanta to visit Sam's adult sister. I desperately wanted to tag along, and I cried and cried when they told me I'd be left out. I don't remember my mother cradling me and telling me it was all going to be okay. She might have, but that's not what I remember.

Instead, I remember that I was on my bed, sniffling and feeling sorry for myself, when she popped her head in. "Hey, let's go see *Grease* at Thruway Shopping Center," she said. "Let's walk there."

Huh? That's eight miles away!

"It's something to do, something different," she said, smiling mischievously. "An adventure."

So that's what we did; we walked to the theater. We stopped on the way and got ice cream. Ever since then, *Grease* is one of my favorite movies—not for the movie itself, but because it reminds me of how my mom could create memories. To this day, I get choked up thinking about the day Mom and I walked to the movies. And if *Grease* is playing on a cable channel, I'll phone her right away and we'll watch a few minutes together, each of us silent.

Mom instilled in us a willingness to be different. I was an athlete in high school, yes, but I was also vice president of my senior class, and I acted and danced in school and community theater productions. I remember preparing for our 1982 production of *West Side Story*, my all-time favorite play. One moment, I was in the gym lifting weights getting ready for football season; the next, I was with Mom at the mall, buying a dance belt for the play. You know what a dance belt is? It's like a jock, only it's more of a thong, and it pulls everything up. I'd wear a jock for football and a dance belt for our play—and, because of the confidence instilled in me by Mom, I could laugh off the good-natured ribbing of my gridiron teammates when they saw the dance belt in my locker.

So often, growing up is about conforming to labels: There are the jocks, the nerds, the brainiacs. We never thought like that. That came from Mom, but she wasn't alone. I had a de facto second mom: my big sister Susan.

When I came along—the baby—Susan dropped Stephen and Synthia like a bad habit and doted on me. She and I have always had a different kind of closeness than that which I share with Synthia and Stephen. We get each other. Like me, she's type A, hard-driving. And she might be the smartest person I know. Growing up, she was our mother hen. She is fiercely loyal and will speak her mind to anyone in defense of her siblings. During my sixteen-day hospital stay in September 2013, a medication I was taking caused my vital signs to crash, and the catheter they'd placed in my manhood was creating severe discomfort. (Guys, anyone who says that a catheter *there* won't hurt hasn't had the procedure done to them, okay?) I didn't have the energy to even speak, which is why patients need strong advocates with them in the hospital. It's not that anybody is trying to hurt you; it's just that you need someone to say, "Hey, Doc—*now!*" And I had Susan as my voice.

"You need to listen to him," she told one of the doctors, whom I didn't really know: She was on the team of my regular docs. "He's not dramatic and he doesn't make stuff up. So if he's saying something is really bothering him, it's really bothering him."

"I know," the doctor said. "I've been taking care of your brother all week—"

"I've been taking care of him his whole *life*," Susan pointedly replied. Silently, I was like, *You go, girl! Give 'em hell!*

Susan has been a very successful corporate executive. Once, when she momentarily fell on some hard times, she asked me for

40

money. And I could tell she hated it. I just stopped her. "Here's why you need to stop," I said. "I'm going to help you, and it doesn't begin to stack up to the ways you've helped me in life." When I was younger and struggling to make it as a TV reporter, she helped me with money. It's what family does. Even today, Susan is the person I call when I need advice or simply need a good cry.

Synthia is the saint of the four of us. She's the most spiritual. We're all Christians, but her sense of values and morals is stronger than that of anyone I've ever met. Growing up, she was a goody-two-shoes, but an athletic, *ass-kicking* goody-two-shoes. She was a superb high school athlete—a three-sport star every year. She played soccer for Anson Dorrance at UNC at the beginning of that program's dynastic run and won two national titles there. She's a former Secret Service and ATF agent and is now chief of a firehouse in Charlotte, North Carolina.

She may be pious, but she's tough. And that was true growing up; Synthia was a protector. She was respected in the neighborhood. The McCarthy boys lived down the street from us. They were some tough Irish kids. We'd play with them, but—kids being kids—we'd also fight with them. One day, when I was twelve, I got into it with Jeff McCarthy—who was fifteen, a year older than Stephen. I don't remember why I was fighting him, but I remember just swinging. He was bigger and stronger and he was peppering me with blows, splitting my lip while I flailed away.

Just then, I could hear Synthia before I could see her. The sound of her sprinting down the street signaled to me that the cavalry was on its way, and she arrived with ill intent. She pulled

McCarthy off me and gave him a legendary Benbow Street beat-down. After that, she had her street cred. No one in the neighborhood messed with her again, not even the toughest boys around, John Wayne Kelly and Jesse James Kelly. Yeah, with names like those, how could you not rumble? But even *they* kept their distance from Synthia.

Stephen and I were closest in age, and he was my constant playmate. We used to go over to other kids' houses and leave confused: This was how they played? Because at home, Stephen and I created whole alternative worlds for ourselves. We were constantly improvising, with ongoing characters and elaborate storylines that played out for hours at a time. Today, I view what I do on *SportsCenter* as storytelling—and whatever creative mojo I have doing it can be traced directly to the hours that Stephen and I spent in our bedroom on Benbow Street.

We had the G.I. Joe, Steve Austin, and O. J. Simpson dolls, and we'd borrow one of our sister's Barbies so that, in what may now be seen as a chilling case of foreshadowing, O.J. could have a pretty, blond girlfriend. When we were still in Chicago, Stephen had a crush on a fellow third-grader named Kelly. I just remember she had some sexy eyebrows. Somehow, that turned into "playing Kelly," which meant we'd agreed on a setup—we were both police detectives, Kelly was his girlfriend, and she'd been abducted—and then we'd just go, ad-libbing all the way.

I had an imaginary friend that, for some reason, was named Jane Jane Shittufah. That led to a whole 'nother narrative—we called it playing Jane Jane. Stephen and I would be in one gang and Jane Jane headed the bad guys' gang, which consisted of Midget Moe, his brother Midget Moo, and Coba C.

Years later, I pledged Alpha Phi Alpha, the black fraternity, in my sophomore year at UNC. Stephen had done the same the year before at Western Carolina University. Part of the pledge process was a boot camp, and you were prohibited from smiling. I was like a sphinx—until one day the brothers called Stephen and had him visit to help break my composure. He just walked up to me, leaned in real close, and whispered, "I'm Jane Jane Shittufah," and I fell out, literally slapping my knee. Even today, we talk about Jane Jane and Kelly and how we had O.J. paired off with a Nicole Brown Simpson look-alike while, in real life, he was still married to his first wife.

Not to sound like too much of an old-timer, but when Sydni gets home from school, there's Facebook, her iPhone, and the TV to occupy her mind. I'm a big believer in the value of all those technological advancements, but when I think back to Stephen and me playing in our room for hours on end, I can't help but wonder if something hasn't been lost from those days. After all, there was no Twitter, Nintendo, or even cable TV. If we weren't outside playing sports, we were inside lost in these intricate worlds of our own making, where we were limited only by the elasticity of our imagination.

Stephen and I could be crudely silly together; in fact, I still pull a lot of our old hijinks today. For example, I like to fake fall in crowded places; when you pull it off just right, the expression on bystanders' faces is priceless. I started doing it in seventh grade, falling off our bicycles with my buddy Robby Fox, and it continues today. I was in Laguna with Kristin and Sydni and fell—everyone around us gasped, but Kristin and Sydni, knowing me, just rolled their eyes and kept walking. Even when I'm getting a chemo infusion, when the unsuspecting nurse first puts in the IV line, I fake pass out—it's worth it to see that brief moment of panic in her eyes before she realizes her patient is just a big kid.

I know it seems insensitive today, but when we were kids Stephen and I used to play blind. One of us would put on sunglasses and walk into the grocery store while holding the other's shoulder; the "blind" one would say, "C'mon, man, let me drive—I haven't driven since the incident." Mom and Dad used to kill us for doing it, but we could tell they were secretly amused by it, too.

But it wasn't all just fun and games. Stephen played big brother protector, too. When I was in fifth grade, Stephen was in a different school for seventh grade—nearly two miles away. My nemeses were Gary and Dale—two white boys at the bus stop who we referred to, respectively, as Flatface and Fatface. One day, I got into a fight with one of them. I think it was Flatface. I handled him. The next day, a Friday, it was Fatface's turn. He jumped me and I sent him home with a bloody lip. Another kid told me that when Fatface got home his father upbraided both boys: "You jump on that nigger and whup his ass next time!" he instructed them.

I was heading for a whupping on Monday. I couldn't handle both brothers at the same time. I told Stephen about my dilemma. He seemed not to hear me. After school on Monday, as the bus rolled up to my stop, Flatface and Fatface rushed off and waited for me on the sidewalk. I shuffled off the bus, resigned, ready to take my beating.

But there, leaning up against a tree, was Stephen. He'd raced nearly two miles after school to get there. When they jumped me, he jumped them, and we commenced kicking those boys' butts. A lady came out of her house and yelled, "Stop doing that! What are you doing?" And Stephen said, "It's okay, ma'am, we're just playing Army!"—as he kneed Fatface in the side of the head.

He'd seemed uninterested when I told him over the weekend what I'd be facing. Yet there he was. Stephen had gone from playmate to hero.

I THINK I FELL so in love with football because it's the one sport where every single play is filled with violence and physicality, and yet you've got your family around you, protecting you. More than any other sport, football is about that Band of Brothers mentality. It's just you and these other guys, and the prevailing ethic among you is: *I'm going to fight for you.*

And it's not just like that in the game. Every single moment of football *practice* is filled with that kind of camaraderie. There's something about the combination of all that violence with all that caring that hooked me. I've never been in the military, but I bet it's similar. The closest thing I've ever felt to football's "one for all and all for one" mentality came in the theater. You work on a production for weeks on end, and there's all this action backstage: set changes, costume changes, running lines. You're in it together, and you're dependent on one another.

When I try to recall what I was thinking and feeling in those first heady moments of my love affair with the game, it wasn't anything about getting a college scholarship or making it to the pros or even experiencing the thrill of competition. It was purer than all that. It was thinking all the time: *I love this.* Running a tight pass route. *I love this.* Throwing a block that frees a team-mate. *I love this.* Coming off the field to the sound of my amped-up teammates slapping my shoulder pads in celebration. *I love this.* And that passion remains just as powerful today. Every single time I've played catch with a football, the reason I've had to stop was either it was time to go, practice was over, or I had somewhere else to be. I've never felt bored throwing a football back and forth. I've never said to myself, "I don't feel like doing this anymore."

In my second year of football, I started touching the ball more. I was naturally fast, and I played wingback in a wishbone offense. The first touchdown I ever scored came that second year on a 21 trap—I went 15 yards. Here I was in a uniform just like Gale Sayers and Roger Staubach, and I'm scoring touchdowns. Yes, plural: that same game included two more, one from the 26-yard line and the other from the 15.

Man, I was hooked. It felt good inside. I turned into a good wide receiver. I wasn't blinding fast, but I could outrun guys and I ran crisp routes and could catch. There's something magical about how it all comes together, the act of running a route and getting your hands around a spiraling ball that's delivered to the perfect spot at the precise moment you come out of your break.

I played other sports, but nothing held me like football. When I was fourteen, I took tennis lessons from David Lash, a legend-ary coach. He'd taught John Lucas, who had gone on to be the top-ranked collegian and play on the pro circuit while also being the top pick in the NBA draft. Lash told me I had a lot of poten-tial in tennis. But I kept telling him I loved football. "You'll never make it in football," he finally said. "You're too small."

I never went back to him. You're going to tell me you don't think I can play football? Man, I don't got no time for you. I'll *show* you.

When I enrolled at Reynolds High School in 1980, I was in the weight room one day when one of the football players was trying to bench-press 110 pounds and was having trouble with it. He was a little guy, maybe 150 pounds. I started laughing at him. "Man, you on the football team and you can't bench 110?" I said.

"You making fun of me?" he said. "What's your name?"

"Stuart Scott."

"You Stephen's brother?" He smiled. And so it was that I met my best friend in life by calling him out on being a weak-ass brotha.

Fred Tindal ultimately mastered that weight and grew to be a solid 280-pounder. To this day, we speak multiple times a week, despite the fact that he's in Abu Dhabi working a civilian job after retiring as a major from the Air Force. He named his daughter Sydney, and then two months later, by weird coincidence, I followed with my Sydni. "You know people are going to think we coordinated this so we could have daughters with the same name," I said to Fred.

"People are not going to believe this," he said. Then we looked at each other: *Who cared what other people thought?*

Every year for the past decade we've met for Daddy-Daughter Week, just us and our daughters, and those weeks are among the best memories of both our lives. One year we went to Aspen; another, Nantucket.

You know how best friends seem to always share an inside joke, even if they can't really define what it is? They just have a sensibility in common and operate together on an altogether different wavelength? That was me and Fred from the start. We were always messing with people, pulling pranks. We'd stage fights—in the library or parking lot we'd seemingly really throw down, gathering a crowd, until we'd let on it was all a fake.

Like me, Fred didn't allow himself to be pigeonholed. Though he played football (his dad made him quit his senior year out of concern for his safety), he was also in the drama club, and acting brought us together as much as football did. We were in *West Side Story*, which is my favorite play because it is both macho and artistic. I was a Shark, and the play took on symbolic meaning for me. As a black kid who'd get into his share of scuffles, I related to being a gang-fighting Shark. But the performance aspect called to me, as well; later, I'd learn some modern dance and do some choreography in college, but this was the first time I'd danced, and it felt very much like football: There was this need inside me to be physically self-expressive, and I just loved everything about the act—including that sense of camaraderie, which Fred was a big part of.

Our love for the arts didn't always mesh well with football. I had to leave practice early four or five times in the run-up to the *West Side Story* production, and I remember our old-school, crew-cutted coach, Doug Crater, wasn't too happy about it. He didn't put up a big fuss—which kind of surprised me—he just grumbled and said, "Okay."

By then I was the captain of our team. I led Reynolds in receiving as a junior, but it was with only 12 catches in a ten-game season. We just didn't throw the ball that much, but neither did anyone else: I was the city's second-leading receiver. Still, there were enough moments that led me to think I could really play this game. We played Greensboro Page, one of the best teams in the state. They featured Haywood Jeffires, who would go on to catch a few hundred passes in the NFL, and Mack Jones, who would star with Haywood at North Carolina State. They beat us 35–21, but I caught an acrobatic touchdown in that game that helped validate me as a receiver.

Meantime, Fred and I were inseparable. We'd hang out in the garage of one of Fred's neighbors, Gilbert Shelton, a kindly older black man. Mr. G would spend the day making bamboo chairs there, and we'd sit around and soak up his wisdom. One day, Mr. G said, "Hey, fellas, you hear that thunder last night?"

"Nah, Mr. G, I didn't hear anything," I said.

"You didn't hear it?" he said. "Goodness, it was loud. It was like: *Boo-yah!*" He yelled it so loud, it startled me as if it were real thunder.

Fred started laughing. "How'd that thunder go, again, Mr. G?"

"BOO-YAH!"

And another of our inside jokes was born. On the playground or in our streets, it came to represent a blast of energy. Someone laid somebody out in the secondary? *Boo-yah!* Someone went yard on the diamond? *Boo-yah!* Someone said something about your mama that totally shut you up? *Boo-yah!*

Years later, when the phrase caught on and became part of my national identity, I was as surprised as anyone else, because I was just talking the language of my youth, one Fred and I had developed.

Because of my passion for the game, I was driven to excel on the football field. When *Rocky* came out in 1976, one of my sisters was dating Bruce Hopkins, a defensive tackle at Wake Forest. Number 99. He gave me the sound track to *Rocky*, and from then on I'd lift weights every day in my room, blaring Bill Conti's inspiring theme song. Today, my dad says that when he'd see me pumping iron after school with the words "gonna fly now . . ." filling the air, he knew that I'd do whatever I needed to do in order to accomplish my goals.

Which doesn't mean there weren't setbacks. In the spring of my senior year, I was diagnosed with keratoconus, a disease of the cornea. I had to have a cornea transplant; the first one didn't go right, so I had to have a second transplant shortly thereafter. Before it, my big sister Susan wrote me the most touching letter. I've misplaced it in recent years, but I remember it saying how much I meant to her and that she'd always be there for me. For years, whenever I'd get down, I'd just reread that letter—and any sense of feeling alone would disappear.

It would be the first of eighteen—yes, you read that right— *eighteen* eye surgeries throughout my life. But even with the transplant, I was going to play football. And my heart was set on playing it at UNC, where my sisters had gone and where Fred was completing his freshman year.

My senior year at Reynolds, I caught another 12 balls—again, among the best totals in the city. I was recruited heavily by three schools: Lenoir-Rhyne University and Catawba College, both of which played in Division II, and Western Carolina University, where Stephen went, which played 1-A ball.

I gave Western Carolina serious thought, but Stephen advised me against it. "You won't like it," he said. The school is in Cullo-whee, North Carolina, and there was a city about seven miles away. Outside that city was a sign that read: "Nigger Don't Let the Sun Set on Your Ass Here." Stephen knew my personality better than anyone. "You'd be getting into a lot of fights here," he told me.

No calls or letters came from Chapel Hill. I knew how good I was, and I couldn't help but think that if we'd only thrown the ball more, if I had 25 catches instead of 12, more schools would have recruited me.

I had a decision to make. Do I go the safe route and attend a Division II school, where I'll no doubt have a shot at meaningful playing time? Or do I go to UNC anyway and try to defy the odds as a walk-on?

That would be the harder thing. But I knew enough to know that the harder thing usually ends up being the most rewarding. UNC, here I come.

CHAPTER THREE

ALPHA MAN

don't think I'm *that* old now, but when you think about it, I attended UNC during the Dark Ages. It was the early eighties. There was no such thing as a cell phone (we had to wait in long lines to use a pay phone to call home), no Internet, and hardly any cable TV. I went on to a career in television, but Fred and I didn't even have a TV in our room.

Fred was a year ahead of me. When I got there, we persuaded his roommate to swap rooms with me—otherwise, the dude was going to have *two* roommates. When I moved in early in my freshman year, that's where we stayed till we both graduated: Ehringhaus Hall, room 021.

So what *did* we do with all our time? Man, we hung out. You remember your college days, right? Our social life consisted mostly of just chillin', a group of kids sitting on lower bunk beds, talking about anything and everything, ordering pizzas late at night. We were, all of us, basking in a newfound sense of freedom. My parents were strict but they didn't sit on me; I had leeway growing up. Nothing like this, however. Suddenly, like so many of my friends, I was making every decision every day for myself. I loved that. We were there to figure stuff out: figure out girls, figure out our studies, figure out who we were. It was like this group project we were all embarking on.

My first week at UNC, I quickly learned that this is what you did: You chilled on the "yard" near the undergrad library or you visited girls in their dorm rooms and just hung out. Fred and I both had girlfriends, and we made a love-song cassette mixtape for when one of us had the room to ourselves with our respective girl. If you came back to the room and heard the mixtape playing through the closed door, you knew to go somewhere else. Later, Fred and I would go over to the girls' dorm rooms and serenade them with our velvety voices, singing everything from Luther Vandross to Billy Ocean.

It was probably the most social I've ever been in my life. Because I'm on TV and I appear comfortable in and around large crowds, a lot of people expect me to be an extrovert. But I've always felt introverted. Recently, Sydni explained to me the difference between the two terms, and it hit home. "Being introverted doesn't have to do with being shy," she told me. "An introvert is someone who, when they're most stressed, gets their energy back by being alone. An extrovert gets recharged by interacting with people."

Smart kid. Wonder where she got that from. I've always felt like an introvert, but I'm not shy or uncomfortable around people. It's just that when I want to recharge, when I need to get my mojo back, when I want to feel at peace, I need to do that alone.

But back then in the early eighties? I had energy to burn. One day, during my first week on campus, I left Fred at our dorm room to visit a classmate. I don't remember her name, but when I got there, her roommate already had a visitor. There, sitting on the bed, all long-limbed, with that sardonic smile the nation was already getting to know, was Michael. As in Jordan.

"Wassup."

"Wassup." That baritone.

Our first conversation. It would be pretty lacking in substance. We talked mostly to the girls. Sports didn't come up. I'd always been a die-hard Carolina fan; I hadn't even applied anywhere else after rejecting those football scholarships. Growing up, Stephen and I used to cut out the bottom of a plastic cup, tape it above our bedroom door, and have some simulated hoops wars—and I'd always be the Tar Heels. We'd keep stats and standings, and, because of our ferocious dunks, the paint above the door chipped away. My favorite point guard—to this day—was the seventies' Tar Heel Phil Ford, who controlled the tempo of a game like no one I'd seen before and who sported a huge, cool Afro.

But though I was a Tar Heel fanatic, I wasn't starstruck by Michael Jordan. He was, by then, already well known. Two years before, as a freshman, he'd led UNC to the national title. Had it been Phil Ford in that dorm room, someone I grew up emulating on the playground, I might have been in awe. But from the moment I met him, Michael was a peer who was still free enough to be a regular kid on campus. We joked around in that dorm room, and then, within a week, it happened again. I went to visit a different girl. In I walked, and there was MJ, wearing Tar Heel blue, talking to her roommate.

"You again?" I said, shaking his hand.

"We gotta stop meeting like this, man," he said, both of us laughing.

From then on, I'd see him often. He lived in Granville Towers, where the basketball players stayed, but he dated a girl on

South Campus, so he'd ride his bike over there all the time. Or I'd see him in the poolroom at the student union. Just one of the guys. At Woollen Gym, I played a few games of pickup basketball with him. If you were on Michael's team, you knew you'd be playing for a while. You ended up on a team playing against him, and it meant you'd be sitting back down right quick.

We were never tight friends, but always friendly. Whenever I'd run into him on campus, I'd be struck by how happy he seemed. Little did I know that, while I was basking in my newfound sense of freedom, those days would be among the last that Michael could enjoy his, that his life would soon be engulfed by a fame it's hard for any of us to wrap our heads around.

IT'S BEEN THIRTY YEARS since those carefree days on campus, and it feels like a lifetime of conversations with Michael Jordan followed. For a time, quite literally: In the mid- to late nineties, Michael would only do the ESPN Sunday Conversation with me. I knew then that that had more to do with our alma mater than me. Michael's loyalty to the school was such that, when he could, he was going to reward fellow Tar Heels. And I'm sure he was more comfortable with me since we had a history together.

Our conversations through the years—whether on the air, at charity golf tournaments, or in VIP rooms in hot and sweaty clubs—didn't go deep. We'd talk sports or, if in a group, bust on each other. Everyone who knows Michael knows he's guarded with his feelings. He's the antithesis of his buddy Charles Barkley—and that's why their friendship works.

Charles and I have had some deep talks over the past couple of decades, much more intense than anything I've ever shared with Michael. For all his advertised toughness, Charles is an introspective and sensitive soul. He texts me every few weeks, just to see how I'm doing. When I was first diagnosed, he called me to say: "Hey, boy, if you need someone to come to Connecticut and hold your hand, I'm there." Taelor was born on his birthday— February 20—and they call each other every year. In 2005, when Taelor turned ten, their birthday fell on the night of the NBA All-Star Game in Denver, where I rented a room and threw a birthday bash for the two of them. Charles and I have bonded over our roles as Dad—his daughter, Christiana, is in her mid-twenties. At the specter of his daughter bringing home a young suitor, Charles said: "I feel like saying to him, 'I know what you're here to do to my daughter.'" Imagine the terror that kid would feel!

Michael would never be so raw. Until, that is, we spoke last year at his annual golf tournament, which I've played in every year since 1997. We were sitting side by side, two aging alums. We started talking about our kids, and the dude came alive in a way I hadn't seen since those dorm room and pool hall encounters three decades ago.

"How you doing with the twins?" I asked, referring to his newborns.

"Man, it's just great," he said, that familiar baritone bouncing with giddiness. "I get up every time. Every time Yvette gets up in the night, I get up because I want to feed them, and I'm giving them their milk in the middle of the night and changing their diapers. I just love it."

He asked after Sydni and Taelor. Meantime, his older boys, Jeffrey and Marcus, were making their way around the banquet hall. Jeffrey came over. I've been around Michael when people approach him in crowds, and there is, by necessity, a look he gives people: polite but detached. But as Jeffrey approached, everything stopped. The outside world melted away. He rose and threw himself into an embrace with his boy. Meantime, Marcus was glad-handing his way across the room.

"Man, Marcus is the mayor," I said of Michael's second oldest. I follow Marcus on Twitter—he's a social guy and he's good at it. "He's the star of the family."

"I know he is," Michael says. "He knows everybody."

As the night wore on, countless people approached, wanting their picture taken with Michael or just to shake his hand. He was polite and generous. At one point, he sat back down and leaned over to me.

"You ever get tired of all this, man?" he said, referring to the demands his public persona has placed on him.

Surprised, I said, "Dude, I am, like, nowhere near *your* level."

He thought for a moment. "I don't hate it," he said. "Sometimes, it's just tiring. You just have to do it."

"Yeah, you just have to accept it as part of the deal," I said. He nodded. I realized I hadn't asked after his daughter. "By the way, how's Jasmine?"

"Great, man," he said, instantly beaming again. "She just graduated college. She's got a job working with the Bobcats now."

There we were, a couple of middle-aged guys just talking about our kids. It was our most human conversation after thirty years of talking about sports. And that's when I got to thinking.

I've been lucky enough to have interviewed and have ongoing relationships with the three most iconic African-American men of the modern era: Michael, Tiger Woods, and Barack Obama. And as cool as that may sound, the most meaningful interactions I've had with all of them have been when we talk about our kids. Those are the conversations I remember—not the ones about a jump shot, a par-five, or some policy prescription for the economy. No, the moments of real connection that have stayed with me have always been about what *really* matters.

I'd see Tiger a lot back in the day. I didn't see or speak to him for probably a year and a half after all that messiness in his private life went down. He understandably retreated into himself and focused on getting his life in order. Meantime, I cringed at how the media covered that story. I often felt embarrassed to be part of this media machine that exploits sports stars' private troubles. The idea that Tiger somehow let *us* down is pure bull. He didn't betray *us*. He had some problems in his marriage. It happens to people every day—but they're not forced by a hyperventilating media pack to make public statements of contrition. Anyway, the first time I saw him after all that, it was at a public event, and his eyes lit up when he saw me. Moments after we embraced, he was searching for his phone. Before I knew it, I was watching video of his two kids—one of them swinging a golf club. I'd never seen him so happy, just being a dad.

When I see Tiger now, he seems content. Most men—athletes or not—don't go out of their way to gush about their kids. I do, as do my closest guy friends. But we're a rarity, and it's as though, in recent years, we've welcomed Tiger into our club. He is just so into being a dad.

I suspect that has something to do with becoming a single dad. Tiger's always loved his kids, as I did, but when you're no longer married, suddenly your time with them becomes all the more precious. And you no longer have that parenting partner to fall back on, so you have no choice but to be selfless. To wit: I didn't play Tiger's celebrity charity golf tournament three years ago because it fell on a weekend I was scheduled to have Sydni and Taelor—and those dates were sacrosanct.

The busiest man I know, the guy with the most pressure on him, seems to have this parenting thing all figured out. I was in Paris in 2008 with the kids and my ex-wife, Kim—post-divorce, we'd still often travel together as a family—when ESPN called; candidate Obama, a hoops fanatic, consented not only to being interviewed by me but to going *mano a mano* with me on the court. How could I say no? I asked my girls for permission to fly back to the States to do the interview. Sydni, then eight years old, had one condition: that, after it was done, I come back to Paris and carry her around the City of Lights on my shoulders for an entire day. Done.

I had met Obama once before. He was on the campaign trail near my home, doing a meet and greet in a neighbor's house. He saw me and smiled. "We've spent a lot of nights together in hotel rooms, you and I," he said. The first thing he ever said to me.

That time, we ended up talking about our girls. I told him that Taelor, the elder, was into shopping, but Sydni not so much. "Just wait, man," he said, smiling knowingly. "Trust me. Been there. They'll *both* get there."

When we squared off on the hardwood, I quickly learned that the dude is a serious basketball player. Classically trained. Nice lefty crossover, smooth pull-up jumper. You can tell he's gotten good coaching and knows the sport. I, on the other hand, am a football player. I'm athletic, but he's a better basketball player than I am. Early in our game, he drove and I fouled him pretty hard. It's the first time I've ever fouled someone on a basketball court who had a Secret Service agent hovering nearby. "You know he's going to be president someday," the agent joked after the hit.

The only way I could stay in the game was to rough him up, to play extra-physical. And with an armed guy nearby, I was kind of dissuaded from amping up the aggressiveness too much. But I'm not making excuses. Even if I had bodied him up more, I couldn't have beaten him—I could have only extended the game a little longer. He took me to Barack's House of Pain, 7–3.

Afterward, we chatted again about our girls. He did a twenty-second video message to my daughters: "Taelor and Sydni, I'm with your dad, playing basketball, and I just wanted to let you know he's thinking of you and is proud of you."

Subsequently, on two separate occasions, I had friends who would be seeing him, and I told them to ask him about our game. Both times, Obama responded the same way. "Oh, yeah," he said. "I handled him."

I handled him. You know who else would have said something like that? Michael. In fact, I remember reading during a particularly stressful time in the '08 campaign, when all seemed hopeless and lost, that Obama told his campaign aides, "Just give me the ball. I'm like Jordan." There *is* a certain similarity there, a common swagger. Not to mention a shared wiseass nature—with a biting edge.

In 2012—four years after his beatdown of me—I saw the president at a fund-raising event in Tampa. Taelor went with me. After he spoke, we made our way across the crowded room to say hello. He saw us and called out, loud enough for many to hear: "Stuart, did you stretch?" He had that same sardonic smirk Michael gets when he's getting on you. "How are your hamstrings feeling from when I beat you? They recover yet?"

"Thanks a lot, Mr. President," I said, laughing. "You're going to talk trash about me in front of my daughter? Thanks a lot."

We took an official photo with him, but then I whipped out my cell phone and asked the Secret Service agent to take a picture of the three of us. "I can't," the agent replied.

"Of course you can," the president said. "Take a picture of my man and his daughter and me."

I cherish that picture, but—as in my relationship with Michael and Tiger—what I cherish more is that we share common values. My friends who don't have kids don't understand. As much as I love Kristin, my parents, and my siblings, the fact is that Taelor and Sydni are really the only two people in my lifetime whom I loved with all my heart and soul *the exact moment I first laid eyes on them.* It's instantaneous and it's overwhelming. And, without ever necessarily coming out and saying it, the constant thread in all of my interactions with three of the biggest names in recent history is really a shared acknowledgment of how life-changing, and life-affirming, it is to have kids.

SOME YEARS AGO, I read the following quote from Spike Lee and thought instantly of my time at UNC: "It comes down to this," he said. "Black people were stripped of our identities when we were brought here, and it's been a quest since then to define who we are."

In some small way, I recognized my own experience in Spike's description. Clearly, I was born here, and nothing nearly as traumatic as slavery or even overt institutional racism had ever happened to me when I was growing up in Winston-Salem. But we never fully fit in, with either the whites or the blacks. It was when I got to college that all that seemed to change. There, I grew to embrace my racial identity at the same time that I reveled in the wonders of diversity. The result is that, today, I am comfortable among any group, anywhere. Today, I never feel like I don't belong wherever I am.

UNC was maybe 12 percent black at the time, but the number felt much higher than that. There were times when it felt like an all-black campus. We'd have all-black parties at Great Hall or you'd sit on the wall outside the library, where the brothas would hang, and there was this feeling of belonging that I'd never experienced before.

Even today, how many people do you pass during the course of one day on the street? Hundreds, right? Black men, when we pass each other, we tend to nod to each other. You see a brother and give a flick of the head, as if to say, *What's up?*—especially if you happen to be in a crowd of white people. This isn't about being separate; it's about acknowledging a shared common ground.

I know, because it doesn't just happen with race. It happens with cancer patients, too. We don't have to talk about how jacked up chemotherapy is and how much cancer wipes you out or how tough it is on our loved ones. Just looking at and hugging one another acknowledges all that; it says, *I get it*. Same with black folk; I don't have to sit and discuss with a brother how tough it is to be a black man. I just nod and he just nods, and we've established a fleeting common connection.

At UNC, I discovered this camaraderie—which, previously, had been the feeling that attracted me to football and the theater. A sense of belonging to something bigger than myself. And that feeling really came together for me when I pledged Alpha Phi Alpha in my sophomore year.

Alpha is the oldest black fraternity in the Greek system, founded in 1906 at Cornell University. Its motto is "First of All, Servants of All, We Shall Transcend All," and its stated goal is "manly deeds, scholarship, and love for all mankind." It's about brotherhood, scholarship, and service. It builds leaders. Through the years, it's been at the forefront of our country's social movements, addressing everything from apartheid to AIDS to urban housing. We had a saying: "Not every great man is an Alpha, but every Alpha is a great man." Among the great Alpha men are Martin Luther King Jr., Thurgood Marshall, and Andrew Young.

But those names, as great as they are, aren't what did it for me. No, I had long yearned to be an Alpha because Stephen was an Alpha—he'd pledged two years before at Western Carolina. And because Synthia had pledged Alpha Kappa Alpha, which is Alpha Phi Alpha's sister sorority. And because Fred was an Alpha, having pledged as a sophomore, my freshman year. I'd watched Fred go through the grueling pledge process—and it *was* tough. But it didn't scare me off.

Pledging an African-American frat is different; I think it's fair to say it's physically and emotionally harder than pledging all other fraternities. You have to keep up on your own studies while at the same time committing Alpha history to memory—instant recall, even. Because there just might be times when you're having to do push-ups with a stack of books on your back and a Brother shouting nonsensical epithets in your ear while you're expected to recite chapter and verse on Alpha's historic legacy.

When you pledge, you're called a Sphinxman. There were twelve of us in our pledge class—some pretty prominent names today—and we'd march in a straight line around campus. There were strict behavioral rules: You had to maintain a "Sphinx-like" expression, you couldn't eat sweets, and you couldn't socialize.

Well, you *could* do anything you wanted to—you just had to hope you didn't get caught by a Brother. One night, I was discovered in a girl's dorm room. It was completely innocent—we were just studying. But that didn't matter. I wasn't supposed to be there.

The next pledge session, I was ready to get my butt wrung out in front of my fellow Sphinxmen. Only something else happened, and it has provided a lesson I carry with me to this day. I was seated in a plush leather chair and treated like some kind of deity. Brothers hovered around me, giving me candy bars, cupcakes, and Coca-Cola—all normally prohibited. The only caveat was I had to watch my linemates get battered—right in front of me. While the Brothers plied me with sweets, they got all over my comrades, in their faces, while I watched, helpless, knowing

I was the cause of my Brothers' distress. It was a brilliant move by the Brothers, having much more of an impact than if they had just given me the business.

It was a powerful lesson. If you mess up, I realized, you're not just messing things up for yourself—you're letting down your family. I learned discipline that night, and I learned that there are other people in this world whose lives are affected by my actions. That night, I learned to never let down anyone who depends on me.

Once an Alpha, I became the Step Master of our wildly popular step shows. Stepping is a type of percussive dance that draws on everything from gymnastics to break, tap, and African tribal dancing; it's a precise, thrilling performance. Stephen and Synthia could both step their butts off, so there was no way I wasn't going to work hard and excel at it, too.

From Alpha, I got what I'd gotten from football and the theater: a sense of belonging, a dawning realization that—this thing you're doing? It's exactly what you're *supposed* to be doing. It's *who* you are.

But that doesn't mean I was done with football. I'd arrived at UNC still determined to walk on to the Division I football team, even though, during my senior year of high school, I had that corneal implant and my eye doctor forbade my playing football until I recovered. Today, after a corneal implant, you'd be good to resume activities like football within a month. Then, recovery included many months of nonaction.

Come sophomore year, I was wrestling with whether to try out. I knew I'd be pledging Alpha. Would going for both only guarantee that I would half-ass each? And, besides, I had to level with myself: A walk-on would probably not see much playing time. No matter how well I played, I'd likely always be behind the scholarship guys.

It wasn't Division I football that held allure for me, after all; it was the game itself. And Carolina had an awesome club football team. We played Division III schools, the Marine Corps, North Carolina State's club team, and Division I-AA schools like South Carolina State and Charleston Baptist College. The quality of play was good, like a cross between semi-pro ball and junior varsity.

I played for three years. We played on Sundays and practiced three or four times a week. I played wideout and cornerback and broke my ribs twice in my senior year—but wore a flak jacket so I didn't miss a game. That year, I took it to Appalachian State: 7 catches, 150 yards, 2 touchdowns. The best part? Even though I wasn't much of a party animal, I'd been out till six a.m. the night before. All those coaches who tell athletes to refrain from extra-curricular activities? Had I known how I'd play after an all-nighter, I might have made that my regular regimen.

Club football was a lot of fun, but I have to admit, I still yearned to find out how I'd do with the big boys on varsity. A lot of the football players lived at Ehringhaus, and one day a bunch of them were playing pickup touch on the field adjacent to our dorm. I joined up, and what transpired led to one of the most satisfying days of my life.

I was playing with guys like Kelvin Bryant, who'd later become a standout running back for the Philadelphia Stars in the USFL and the Washington Redskins in the NFL; Earl Winfield, an all-ACC receiver; and Larry Griffin, who would go on to play in the Pittsburgh Steelers defensive backfield. It was just touch, but everybody was going all-out. And I balled up with those guys. I wasn't the best player on the field, but I more than belonged on it. I scored three touchdowns in that game. Walking off, I remember thinking, *I could have done this.*

But had I done it, who knows if my college experience would have been as well-rounded and rewarding as it was? In high school, I was dead set on playing football in Carolina blue. Funny how things turn out. Who was it that said life is what happens when you're busy making other plans?

I MET THE FEMALE me in an Interpersonal Communications class my junior year. And Barbara Lee met the male version of herself in me. Most Southern girls are bouncy and sweet and demure. They're raised to refrain from speaking their minds, lest they offend. Barb? Hardly any of that applied to her.

Barb wasn't warm and fuzzy—unless you got to know her. I've often thought there's a serious double standard in American culture. Men who are serious and aren't afraid to speak their minds are called great leaders. Women with the same traits are called shrill or, worse, bitches. Barb isn't a bitch—but she's a serious person who won't bat her eyelashes and play smaller than she is just to fit in. We were kindred spirits from the start. We got each other. There was never so much as a flirty word between us. But I knew instantly that here was a lifelong friend.

Through the years, we've been there for each other. We both had daughters within two months of each other, so the phone lines between us were constantly buzzing with parenting talk.

We cried on each other's shoulder when we both went through divorces. When I got sick, she didn't ask what I needed. She'd had loved ones battle cancer and she knew what to do. Once, while I was in the hospital, knowing that when I got home it would be a chore to climb the stairs, she hired a crew of workers and turned my ground-floor storage room into a den so cool, the moment I saw it I felt like I'd been hanging out in it forever. During my hospital stay in September 2013, again without asking, she chartered a plane and flew my parents out to see me—and she put them up. She knew I'd need an assistant after I got sick, so she took it upon herself to interview all candidates and hire one, warning each candidate: "He's not mean; he's just not very talkative. He's all business."

Funny, I could have said the same about her.

I enjoyed that Interpersonal Communications class, but the best thing about it was that it gave me Barb. My second favorite class was Introduction to TV Production, which I also took junior year. I still didn't know what I wanted to do with my life, but I knew I liked TV. In that class we wrote, lit, and directed broadcasts. Writing scripts, planning shots: This was kinda cool.

The first piece I produced was of *Soul Train* impresario Don Cornelius interviewing Tina Turner. Fred was looking all Super Fly playing Don Cornelius, and we convinced a girl named Jeanette to wear a short leather miniskirt and play Tina. I still remember the music underneath—"What's Love Got to Do with It"—building to a climax as the camera slowly panned up Tina's long legs.

The other video I did was a faithful rendition of the scene in *Rocky IV* when Rocky tries to talk Apollo Creed out of fighting the Russian behemoth Ivan Drago. Fred—what a trouper—played Apollo, and our buddy Skee, a Stallone look-alike, did a dead-on Rocky.

I loved learning how to edit. Something that once only lived in my imagination now actually . . . existed, because I created it. I miss editing packages to this day. Before going to ESPN, I won an award for editing together Orlando Magic highlights to the sound of C+C Music Factory's "Everybody Dance Now." There was something thrilling about taking a concept from birth to fruition.

Despite my enthusiasm for editing, I was still searching for what would become my lifelong passion. That changed on May 20, 1986. That was the first day of my summer internship at WTVD in Durham, the ABC affiliate.

I thought I'd basically be photocopying scripts and fetching coffee for the anchors and reporters, but that day the assignment desk sent me out on a story. Shaw University, an all-black school in Raleigh, was having a press conference to address its serious financial issues. Along with a cameraman, I was to cover the event.

Of course, I wasn't going to be on camera. My job was to interview people there so that a sound bite could run on-air that night. When I got back to the newsroom, the producer told me to write up a V.O. bite—a voiceover. I'd done that in our TV Production class. So I sat at an ancient typewriter—remember those?—and pounded out a lead-in to the bite. *Pretty cool,* I thought. *They're having me practice my writing.*

But then the producer came by, looked at it over my shoulder, and said, "Okay, now go show it to Larry."

Gulp. Anchorman Larry Stogner was—and still is—the dean of Durham broadcast journalism. I doubted that he had the time to read my script, so I approached his desk timidly.

"Mr. Stogner, my name is Stuart Scott. I started my internship today," I stammered. "Wanted to show you a V.O. bite."

Larry Stogner seemed like a casting director's *idea* of an anchorman—the perfectly coiffed shock of frosted hair, the deep voice. He slowly looked up from his desk and took the paper from my trembling hand as he put his glasses on. I watched him read. He was looking down at that paper for what seemed like ten minutes, but was probably thirty seconds. He crossed out one word. And then he said:

"All right, thank you, Stuart."

And he flipped the page into the box on his desk that held the scripts for on-air that night. I remember thinking, over and over: *That's going to be a news story. A real news story.*

Later I called my mom and dad, and they heard their son hyperventilating: "When Larry Stogner reads a story tonight about Shaw University, those are my words!" I blurted out. "I wrote that!"

Larry Stogner read *my* words that night on television—the first day of my internship. And I was hooked. This was what I wanted to do.

Today I see Larry Stogner every year at the Jimmy V golf tournament, and I always make it a point to tell him how indebted I am to him. I was just some black kid in the newsroom; he didn't have to take an interest, but he did. And he imparted what was for me a lifelong lesson: the importance of writing.

I tell young people all the time that it doesn't matter if your voice isn't deep or if you're rocking a plaid leisure suit. If you can write, you have a future. Now, I don't mean using flowery, big words to show how smart you are. I mean reading a newspaper article and rewriting it so it can be read in twenty-five seconds. I used to do that every day: practice my writing.

When I got to ESPN, almost all of the other talent had grown up with a common goal: to get to ESPN. Their role models were Boomer and Craig Kilborn and Olbermann. They'd had mentors in the business along the way. But I had never dreamed of one day hosting *SportsCenter*. In college, I didn't even watch TV, let alone faithfully follow the Worldwide Leader. My role models were iconic athletes, people like Muhammad Ali and Walter Payton.

Until my internship, I didn't have mentors in the news business. But at WTVD, I had plenty—and I soaked up as much knowledge as I could. Stogner continued to give me opportunities to prove myself. Denise James was a nightside news reporter who let me shoot stand-ups that I could use on my résumé tape.

Denise, who went on to be a reporter in Philadelphia, was so cool to this intern. She was doing a story on young people having heart attacks and asked if I wanted to be on-camera, hooked up to an EKG. I said sure. When she cut the tape, as footage rolled of me being tested, she said, "Stuart Scott is a twenty-year-old college student in good shape . . ." But I was about to turn twenty-one within a month, and I sheepishly asked if she could refer to me as twenty-one instead.

"But why?" she asked, no doubt more used to people lying in the other direction about their age.

"I don't know," I said, a bit shyly. "Twenty-one is just cooler." No doubt, I was thinking of how it would play with the ladies.

And she did it—because her intern asked her to. The whole staff seemed to take me under its collective wing. One night that summer there was a party for all the twentysomethings on staff, and I was invited. Rick Williams was a news reporter who would go on, like Denise, to the Philadelphia market, and he engaged me in conversation over a couple of beers as if I were his equal. Stogner, James, Williams, photographers like Ron Savage and Steve Denny—who blocked for Phil Simms at Morehead State back in the late seventies—they were all nice to me when they didn't have to be. That stuck with me, and I haven't forgotten it when I relate to interns to this day.

So now I knew what I wanted to do. Little did I know that deciding on a career path would be the easy part. There were hardly any sports reporter jobs open, so, given my experience as Denise's intern, I set my sights on news-reporting positions.

In advance of spring break my senior year, I sent out twenty-seven résumé tapes to small-market stations up and down the East Coast. When school let out for spring break, my friends hightailed it down to Florida for one last fling as a collegian. I was tempted, but someone at WTVD had advised me not to follow up my tape to stations with a phone call asking for an interview; instead, the advice went, just call the news director, say you're in town, could you stop by? Ten minutes later, you just show up! I loved the aggressiveness of that play. So I recruited Stephen for a road trip, and we drove up and down the coast, basically cold-calling TV stations all the while.

We went to Savannah, Augusta, Charleston, Little Washington, Wilmington. One by one, the rejections came until they all blurred into one another. The best—and by best, I mean most traumatic—came when I got back to UNC. I was sitting at my desk in my dorm room late one afternoon. I had sent a tape to the news director at WITN in Little Washington, North Carolina, and now I was following up with a phone call. I got through directly.

"I was just wondering what you thought of my tape," I said.

He said, and I can hear it today as clear as if I'd recorded it: "I'll be honest with you—you suck, and you'll never make it in this business."

For years I remembered this guy's name, because I used it for fuel. But it escaped me a few years back, once I didn't need to prove anything to him anymore.

I remember the way the evening's fading sunlight was streaming through my window when I hung up. I was now officially 0 for 27. All the negative self-talk came in waves: *Would I ever get a job? Maybe I do suck.* The tears started to flow, turning to gasping sobs. For twenty minutes, I sat there, wallowing.

And then, like Ali when Frazier knocked him down with that good-night shot in the fifteenth round of their first fight—you could tell it wasn't his legs lifting him off that canvas as much as his heart—I summoned something from within. I stopped myself. Enough with the self-pity, I thought. And then I said out loud: "I'm going to prove that sonofabitch wrong."

CHAPTER FOUR

GOTTA BE ME

onja. Sonja would know what I should do.

It was June 1987, and my streak of rejections had finally been broken—I had a job offer. So why was I undecided about taking it? Because it hardly paid a living wage, that's why. This wasn't back in the days of black-and-white TV, after all—and they were expecting me to work for $175 a week?

Bob Howick was the anchor and news director at WPDE, the ABC affiliate in Florence, South Carolina. He came off as a cranky, grizzled veteran of broadcast news. I'd later learn that beneath the tough exterior was a kind man. I'd met him some weeks before, when my dad accompanied me to Florence for an interview at the station. Howick was looking to hire a reporter for his Myrtle Beach bureau, which was about fifty miles from the station. "You know, I like you," Howick barked at me. "But you're not ready for this. You'd be all by yourself. You don't have the experience to make that work."

I'd heard that song and dance before. "If anything comes up, I'll let you know," he said. Yeah, right. I bet you say that to all the guys. I was silent on our ride home.

But two weeks later Howick did call. "We have an opening in Florence," he said. "News reporter. I want to offer it to you."

That's when I heard the $175 figure. That's less than $10,000 a year. Even though it ran the risk of Howick hanging up and finding somebody else, I negotiated. Howick agreed to up the salary to $200 per week. But I still wasn't sold. "Let me think about it," I said.

I really was tempted to say no. So I did what you do when you're young and trying to break into an industry—you seek out advice from those who have been where you are. I called Denise James, who told me the same thing as Miriam Thomas, Larry Stogner's coanchor at WTVD in Durham: "Get your foot in the door."

But I still couldn't get myself to yes. That's when I thought of Sonja.

Sonja Gantt is now an anchor at WCNC, the NBC affiliate in her hometown of Charlotte, North Carolina. She and I had been tight throughout college. She called me her "play brother," and she was my "play sister." We were both broadcasting students, and right after graduation she landed a job at number-one-rated WBTW, the CBS affiliate in Florence. She'd been there a couple of weeks. Sonja would know what I should do, because she was already there, yes, but also because she was uncommonly wise.

Her father was Harvey Gantt, the mayor of Charlotte—the first black to hold that office. In 1990 and then again in 1996, he'd challenge Jesse Helms, North Carolina's racist U.S. senator, and lose in two very close elections. Michael Jordan came under some fire for not endorsing Gantt in either of those elections. When asked about it then, Michael said, "Republicans buy sneakers, too." I really wanted to see Gantt win, and Michael's imprimatur in the 1990s could have made a difference. But years later, Jordan gave a more nuanced and persuasive explanation for his silence: "I supported Harvey Gantt privately," he told *GQ* magazine. "But then it became, 'Okay, why won't you speak out politically?' Well, I'd only be setting myself up for someone to scrutinize my opinions, which were limited, because I never channeled much energy into politics."

In other words, Michael smartly saw the call for him to get involved in politics as a way for the media to knock him off the pedestal upon which it had placed him. Jesse Jackson used to say, "There are tree shakers, and there are jelly makers"; Jesse was the former, Michael the latter. *Both* are necessary.

But back when I was contemplating that offer, Michael was lighting it up in Chicago, and Harvey Gantt was still a couple of years away from challenging Helms. And all I needed was for Sonja Gantt to tell me whether to put my reservations aside and join her in Florence.

"You have to do it!" she squealed when I told her the news. "You have to take this job. We'll go grocery shopping together. We'll eat tuna fish every day."

Florence should have hired her to do its marketing. She made it sound like Shangri-La. All my life, I'd sought out a sense of community: that's what drew me to football, the theater, and fraternity life. Sonja knew this and promised me the same in Florence. There were a ton of young TV reporters in Florence just like us, she said, and we'd all hang out together. When you start at an uncommonly low salary, of course, it's nearly impossible to fully make that up in later years, no matter how well you perform your job. But, Sonja pointed out, that concern didn't really apply in this case. None of us, after all, were going to stay in Florence, only the 103rd biggest market in the country. This was a starter job. Bigger markets down the road promised bigger paydays.

So I moved to Florence. I roomed with Terra Redus, one of the other young reporters. For the first and only time in my life, I had a budget book in which I dutifully recorded every expense. I didn't splurge, and I was never in too much debt. Rent was $315 a month. I bought a 1981 Plymouth Reliant K-car for $1,000, and Sonja turned out to be prophetic: I ate vats of canned tuna. One time, I splurged and bought myself dough to make chocolate chip cookies—only to return home one day to the wafting smell of cookies in the air. "Did you make my cookies, Terra?" I asked.

"No," she said, forgetting the maxim we had all learned from Watergate: Often, the cover-up is worse than the crime.

"How you gonna lie to me, Terra? You ate my cookies," I said. Finally, after a bit more cross-examination, she broke down and confessed.

Every Friday night, a group of us would go to Applebee's— me, Sonja, Terra, and Rick Henry, who was WPDE's sports director and one of my mentors. We were all learning together, and our barroom conversations were as much a part of the apprenticeship as our time in the studio or newsroom. After a few months, I was made weekend sports anchor—while continuing my role as weekday news reporter. It wasn't more money, and it meant I'd have literally no free time, but it was invaluable.

It was a great learning experience because you were expected to be a one-man band. The station had only three cameras. I'd take a Betacam with me out in the field and shoot all my own material. How do you shoot a stand-up of yourself? I learned very quickly. You take the light pole, run it up to six feet, position it to where you're going to stand, focus on it with the camera, hit Play, move the light pole, and stand in its place—*holla!* You're recording your own stand-up.

I worked at WPDE for eleven months. In the summer of 1988, at all of twenty-three years old, I made a quantum leap. WRAL in Raleigh—competitor of Stogner's WTVD, where I'd interned—was in the thirty-second biggest market in the country. And the work was top-ten quality.

I was the nightside news reporter. But the assignment desk knew of my affinity for sports, so I'd get all these sports-themed stories. That's how I first met Coach Valvano, when he was going through that recruiting scandal at N.C. State. He had me to the house, where we sat out back and talked for hours after the camera was off. I remember thinking, *If this guy is this cool to a reporter when he's going through a scandal, he must be one special dude.* And that's hard to admit when you're a Tar Heel.

Another time, I did a story on a brash Duke law student who, at twenty-two, had become the youngest registered agent in sports. Drew Rosenhaus had gone to undergrad at the University of Miami when the Hurricanes' football program was at its peak; he turned his close connections with players at "the U" into a career. He was then as he is now: loud, unafraid, a slick operator. The conniving character Bob Sugar, played by Jay Mohr in the movie *Jerry Maguire*, is said to be based on Rosenhaus.

The sports department at WRAL consistently won awards, and I learned from them the importance of great photography. I soaked up the wisdom of sports director Bob Holliday and anchor Tom Suiter. But the true stars were sports photographers Jay Jennings and Jeff Gravley.

To this day, Jennings might be the best I've ever seen. Way back in the late eighties, he was doing stuff well ahead of his time. Video montages, with great jump cuts. Real tight shots on a spiraling football, slowed down, NFL Films–style.

Funny, you know how, when I think back on my relationships with Jordan, Tiger, and Obama, the moments that have stayed with me the most are those in which we've talked about our kids? Well, I admired Jay Jennings's work, but my most powerful memory of him had nothing to do with anything he shot. Jay was a great athlete, and we used to have some killer touch-football games. To one, he brought his four-year-old son, Jason. The last play of the game, we kicked off to Jason, who caught the ball, and those of us on the other team went diving over and beyond him, *just* missing him time and again, while he scampered down the sideline for a touchdown, his dad a step ahead the whole time, shouting, "C'mon, Jason, this way! C'mon, man!"

I was twenty-three, but, looking at Jay's pride and Jason's giggling joy, I knew then: *I want this. I can't wait to be a dad.*

Years later, Jason became a news reporter at WRAL. He's now a sports anchor in Tampa, Florida. That circle-of-life stuff is a trip, man.

"THAT IS ONE BIG DUDE," I said, letting out a low whistle. In the same way you remember that awestruck feeling when you first take in the sheer immensity of the Grand Canyon, so it was that I'd always remember first laying my eyes on this hulking behemoth in front of me.

It was 1992, and my photographer and close friend Ricky Scarwid and I were in Chicago for the NBA Pre-Draft Camp leading up to the draft. By now, I was the sports anchor at WESH, the NBC affiliate in Orlando, Florida, having left WRAL in 1990. The Orlando Magic had the first pick in the draft, and everyone knew it was going to be this giant out of LSU, Shaquille O'Neal. We were there to land Orlando's first interview with him.

Now here he was, checking in to his hotel. He was a little hard to miss. Ricky and I approached, and Shaq couldn't have been more accommodating. He had as many questions for us about Orlando as we had for him about basketball.

But mostly what I remember about him was . . . that *size*. I'd seen taller guys but no one *bigger*. That he was also a great athlete and, as it turned out, a charismatic personality made you think early on: *This is something entirely new.*

Shaq's arrival in Orlando was a type of passing of the torch: What had been Mickey Mouse's town now belonged to Shaq. You know how some people are just silly and goofy? Well, Shaq was silly, goofy, and *smart*. But the goofiness is what set him apart. A lot of times, as practice was about to end, he'd break-dance—it's one of the freakiest sights I've ever seen, a 7'1", 300-pound giant dropping to the ground to bust some moves.

Everything Shaq did was newsworthy. Ricky and I were there when he'd take area kids on toy-shopping sprees at the mall, and the story would lead our sportscast. We were there when he made his rap debut with Fu-Schnickens in a song called "What's Up Doc? (Can We Rock?)," and I loved his riff; I remember it to this day. *"Forget Tony Danza, I'm the Boss/When It Comes to Money, I'm Like Dick DeVos,"* he rhymed, referencing the Magic owner. *"Now, who's the first pick? Me. Word is born'in/Not Christian Laettner, not Alonzo Mourning."* It's fair to say Shaq wasn't happy with all the hype Duke's Laettner received when they both were in college.

Even before Shaq's arrival, I loved my time in Orlando. I had never worked in a city that had a pro basketball team. Our sports director, Marc Middleton, was intense. He'd come in in the morning and stay until eleven p.m. Most days, the Magic were our lead sports story. Marc would send us over to Magic practice, and we'd put together an ambitious 1:30 package on the team for that night's broadcast.

Before Shaq, the Magic weren't very good, but they had a great cast of characters. Dennis Scott, who arrived in town when I did, was the purest three-point shooter I've ever seen. Nick Anderson was a streak scorer—and someone who always seemed like he was in a foul mood in the locker room. Years later, I ran into him, and he was laughing and joking around. I remember thinking, *Where was this personality back in the day?* But some days he must have felt the need to put a wall up. Some guys play better with a permanent scowl. Nick was one of them; the Magic back then won a lot of games they shouldn't have simply because Scott or Anderson would get unconscious and go on a roll.

There was also point guard Scott Skiles—the answer, for a time, to a great trivia question: Who holds the record for most assists in an NBA game (30) and most consecutive home runs by a high school baseball player (4)? I was at the game when Skiles set the assist record. He was aware of what he was about to do, and on one play late in the game, he passed the ball to Jerry "Ice" Reynolds—who promptly passed it to another teammate. "Shoot the f'ing ball!" Skiles yelled.

And there was Litterial Green, a backup point guard who could jump outta the gym. One day at practice, he and I held a slam-dunk contest. He won, but I held my own.

When there wasn't a Magic story to pursue, there always seemed to be something interesting worth covering. There was Banana George, the bare-footed legend of the stunt water-skiing circuit, the only person to have skied on all seven continents. There was Brown's Gymnastics and coach Rita Brown, who produced countless gymnastic stars, including Olympians Wendy Bruce and Brandy Johnson. And there was the time I got in the ring with some pro wrestlers for an on-air lesson in the art of body slamming. That took me back in time to Winston-Salem, when Stephen and I would construct a makeshift ring and wrassle—and I'd always be Ric Flair, my hero in the squared circle.

Life was good—on the air and off. I loved the hot weather and the golf. I met my future wife, Kim, just before moving to Orlando. As a flight attendant, she would pop in and out of town. We made some great friends, including Lisa Rayam, one of WESH's anchors. She was married to Lee Norris Rayam, one of those rare souls you meet in life. He was a singer, an actor, an antiviolence community activist, and a mentor. He was program director for the Central Florida Urban League, and he introduced inner-city youth to poetry to divert them from the bad options that waited on every urban corner. Lee Norris and Lisa sang to each other at their wedding, which was incredibly moving. When Kim and I got married, they sang at our wedding.

Meantime, on the air, I was me. I had learned not to try to be something on TV that I'm not. I started to incorporate different parts of my personality—I love sports, and I was going to let that love fly. I remember a couple of times, my news director said to me, "Hey, tone it down a little. Save that stuff for ESPN."

Funny, I wasn't even a big ESPN watcher. Once I got there, I found out that buddies of mine, like Rich Eisen, came of age watching Dan Patrick, Keith Olbermann, and Craig Kilborn every night and dreaming of being on the *SportsCenter* set. I knew who Dan, Keith, and Craig were, but I didn't care about them. I cared about the games. I didn't relate to the guy reading me the scores; I related to the guys doing the scoring.

I was never interested in being like anyone else or having a shtick. A lot has been said through the years about how I brought something of a racial consciousness to sports broadcasting. I was just being myself—talking about sports the way I would with Stephen or Fred. So who I was on-air wasn't conscious or calculated; I was just lucky to end up somewhere—ESPN—where they let you have a personality and be yourself. They smartly weren't interested in the blow-dried automaton that monotonously dictates scores and highlights.

Instead, I was someone who was passionate about sports and wouldn't suppress my feelings—no matter what a news director said. This is *sports*, man; we ain't curing cancer. Now, in retrospect, I can see how that can be viewed in racial terms. After all, the black athlete has long blazed a trail in terms of self-expression.

From Billy "White Shoes" Johnson's end-zone dances to the emergence of the high-five in the late seventies courtesy of baseball's Glenn Burke and the high-flying Louisville Cardinals in college basketball ("Doctors of Dunk"), the black athlete has led the way in terms of on-field celebration. And the suits in the front offices—especially the NFL—have tried to legislate that celebration out of the game. Hey, suits: It's supposed to be fun. That's why they call it a game.

Like "White Shoes," I was going to let my love for these games show. You know what I've never done at a sporting event? Boo. I don't get the whole idea of booing. You're booing someone because they just failed at something? Seriously? Do you know how hard it is to do what they're doing? That they're among the best in the world at what they do?

Too often, sports coverage is the media equivalent of booing. I never want my broadcast to feel like that. I grew up respecting athletes for what they accomplished and trying to understand what life was like from their point of view. If more of the media had that kind of open-minded curiosity, maybe we wouldn't have such "gotcha" journalism today.

I've been criticized for being too chummy with and soft on athletes. That critique is born of a very particular type of journalism: one in which predominantly white, middle-aged writers and broadcasters paternalistically judge young, often black, athletes. I'll ask tough questions, if need be. But they'll be in service of explaining rather than judging. The viewer can then judge for him- or herself.

For example, when Allen Iverson was arrested early in his career for having a concealed weapon in his car, I didn't ask him:

"How do you square what you've done with your responsibility to be a role model to America's youth?" Instead, I asked him: "You just had a beautiful baby girl. What will you tell her about these events?"

And Allen, God bless him, looked at me and spoke from the heart: "I'll tell her her daddy isn't perfect and that I made a mistake," he said. "And that I'm trying to do better every day."

I loved Allen for that answer, because it was real and full of heart. And that's the interviewer's job: to get past all the artifice and all the clichés, and to arrive at something authentic. Allen would have never been so open and vulnerable if I had come at him like I was judge, jury, and executioner.

IN FEBRUARY 1993, ESPN sent producer Gerry Matalon to Florida to do a feature for *Outside the Lines* on Shaq and Orlando, how this small-market town was adjusting to having this gargantuan phenomenon in its midst. Gerry and I would go on to be great friends. He's now senior coordinating producer of on-air talent development at the Worldwide Leader. I had never met him when he asked to interview me for the piece.

We sat down at a game and did the interview. Afterward, Kim had a thought: "Why don't you go ask if you can send him a tape?"

So I went back to Gerry. "If I want to send ESPN a tape, can I send it to you?" I said. "That way, you can take it to whoever you need to, instead of it just sitting in a pile."

He said he'd be happy to. I sent it off and thought nothing of it. Until the phone rang a couple of months later.

"Stuart, this is Al Jaffe at ESPN," a voice said.

I knew who Al Jaffe was—the vice president of talent. I figured it was one of my boys, probably Fred, busting my chops. "Come on, stop playing, man," I said.

"Uh, I don't play," he said. "This *is* Al Jaffe. We're starting up ESPN2, a new network. It'll be young and hip, and we're interested in you for it. We'd like you to come to Bristol for an interview."

The first thing I did was call around to get some intel on ESPN's interview process. A consensus quickly formed: You'd better know your sports. Like, seriously know sports. Like, be able to name at least five players from every Major League Baseball team—and their stats.

So I made a chart comprising the roster of every pro team in every major league, and I committed it to memory. Lord knows how smart I'd be today if I didn't cram my brain with all that useless information back then. In Bristol, Al Jaffe asked, "Can you name me at least five players from every Major League team?"

"Yeah, I think I can."

"Okay," he said. "Give me five Kansas City Royals."

"George Brett, of course," I said. Jaffe nodded. "You've got David Cone and Tom Gordon on the pitching staff. Wally Joyner . . ."

I owed him one more. "And Greg Gagne," I said, resisting the urge to refer to the shortstop as "Boomer" Berman did: "Gagne with a spoon."

There was silence. "Am I right?" I asked.

Jaffe broke into a slight smile. "I don't know," he said.

And with that, Al Jaffe hired me for the forthcoming ESPN2, where I'd be a *SportSmash* anchor, doing five-minute updates of scores and news every half hour. That meant leaving beautiful Orlando for Bristol, which didn't seem to have a whole lot going on in it. But I didn't care. ESPN was a place where on-air talent had the freedom to be themselves. And I was ready for that.

CHAPTER FIVE

BOOMER
BETTER
KEEP UP

At 7:30 on the night of October 1, 1993, a new sports network was born and carried into some 10 million homes: ESPN2, or, as we called it, the Deuce. Today, ESPN2 is hardly distinguishable from ESPN. But back then, it was going to be a whole 'nother thing. It would be a younger, hipper alternative to ESPN, and the signature show, *SportsNight*, would be the new generation's answer to *SportsCenter*. *Sports-Night* had lowercase on-screen graphics and a graffiti-infused theme running through it. We would focus on alternative sports more attractive to a younger demographic—things like snowboarding and mountain biking. That was the plan, anyway.

On that first night, it was not altogether clear we had a success on our hands when anchor Keith Olbermann, curiously wearing a leather jacket, opened the three-hour show by saying: "Welcome to the end of my career."

Afterward, there was a party to end all parties on our Bristol campus. A parade of limos made its way up the Saw Mill River Parkway from New York City. Studio executives, media honchos, and the random celeb made the trek up to sleepy Bristol to mark the dawning of what we hoped would be a new era in sports broadcast journalism. I remember being in the greenroom and seeing Downtown Julie Brown and MC Hammer—this was a few years after Hammer Time, but the dude was still rocking some puffy pants.

A lot has been said and written about that party. Some ESPN staffers pulled all-nighters. I soaked it all in. I recognized the partying for what it was: a big exhale. There had been a lot of tension leading up to the Deuce's debut.

We'd been rehearsing for months, and Olbermann had already threatened to quit many times. He had moved over from *SportsCenter*, where he and Dan Patrick had helped build a brand, and wore that leather jacket on-air, violating the first rule of cool: If you try too hard to be it, you ain't it.

Keith had a reputation for being difficult. I didn't know him well—and still don't. Full disclosure: Suzy Kolber was, and is, a close friend. She came to the Deuce thinking she was Keith's coanchor. Only Keith didn't see it that way and treated her more like a sidekick.

Either way, it wasn't my business. I've never had a feud with a colleague. Every once in a while, I've had words, especially in my first few years at ESPN. One time, I remember going at it with fellow anchor Brett Haber. There's a tradition on the *SportsCenter* set: The anchor who has seniority gets to choose what side of the set he sits on. Well, I'd been at ESPN longer than Brett, but he'd been at *SportsCenter* longer than me. So it wasn't clear who had more seniority, but I deferred to him and sat opposite where I liked to be: on his left, which is the right side of the screen to the viewer. I didn't think I'd care, but we did the show and I was uncomfortable with the camera angle the whole time. The next day, in our show meeting, Brett wasn't there. I told the director, "Hey, man, tonight I'm sitting on the right, 'cause I like that better."

I swear the color drained from his face. "You're going to tell Brett," he said.

"Sure, I'll tell Brett." What was the big deal? I mean, what was Brett going to do? Get mad at me?

Later, I came up to Brett in the newsroom. "Hey, man, I'm going to sit on your right tonight 'cause I don't like the other seat," I said, before turning and walking away.

He pursued me. "Hey, hey!" he called. "Are you asking me or are you telling me?"

I stopped and spun around, and now we were face-to-face. I was in my late twenties, all fire and brimstone. Instead of defusing things and just saying something like "That's just the way it is, man," I stepped up and then brought it down. I got in real tight, nose-to-nose, and whispered, "Telling you." He froze. Issue done. That night I sat where I wanted and Brett was so, so nice to me. Now, today, I don't think I handled that confrontation in a mature way. But I've gotta say: It *was* satisfying. And the bigger point is that Brett and I were cool from then on. I may have been immature, but I knew even then that life's too short to keep alive meaningless feuds and invent silly slights.

As with Brett, whenever I had a toxic conversation with a colleague, it never went beyond that: It was over and we always went back to being professional. It sounds odd, but that's easy to do when you just don't care what others think of you. If someone didn't like me, I was always aware that that was on him or her. Not my problem, dude.

Suzy was more sensitive than that, and she went through a tough time those first six months of *SportsNight*, until Olbermann hightailed it back to *SportsCenter*. Years later, Suzy would show the world what I saw during the early days of the Deuce: that she was a consummate pro. Her character was on full display when, live on-air, a drunken Joe Namath slobbered over her and kept saying "I want to kiss you" in an embarrassing display that quickly went viral.

I remember calling Suzy during that time and telling her, "I'm sorry you went through that; that must have been tough. But it didn't *look* tough on TV—you handled it with total class." What struck me was how compassionate she was toward Joe—not only when I talked to her after the fact but even in the moment, on live TV. She could have made him look even worse, but while interviewing him and throughout the story that followed she was concerned about Joe—he felt awful about the whole thing—and she was consistently classy. That's the Suzy I got to know at *SportsNight*, the Suzy I coanchored with after Keith went back to *SportsCenter*.

So not even six months after ESPN2 debuted, I was coanchoring a show. That excited me, but I wasn't awed. I think that attitude comes from the athlete in me. I didn't think, *Oh, God, this is national TV.* I thought, *All right, let's do this show, man.* You've got to be a little cocky to succeed. I was doing *SportsNight* and also *NBA2Night*. One year, I did a season of *NFL Primetime* with Boomer and Tom Jackson. I remember very vividly, before my first show with Chris Berman, my colleague Rich Eisen asked, "You nervous doing a show with Boomer?"

I like Boomer. I respect Boomer. He's a great talent. All of us on the air owe him 10 percent of every paycheck we get because he's our *SportsCenter* forefather. But nervous? C'mon, man. "I'm not nervous doing a show with Boomer," I told Rich. "He better keep up." I was going to do my thing.

Meantime, on *SportsNight*, we started to hit our stride as a show once we were cut to an hour per night. It's funny, as at many workplaces, there was always a lot of bitching about management at ESPN. Perhaps that's to be expected when your biggest star, Keith, is also the newsroom's complainer-in-chief. But I never went in for that. If he was ticked off about something, that had nothing to do with me. As a black man in the workplace, you keep your head down and don't bother with stuff that isn't your business. Besides, I was new and happy to be there. But more important, I'm an intensely loyal person. And early in my time at ESPN, something happened that led me to understand for the first of many times just what a caring, compassionate company I was working for.

MY WIFE, KIM, and I were awakened by our ringing phone at two a.m. one day in June 1994. On the other end, all I could hear was sobbing and cries of pain. My heart raced. Was it my parents? One of my siblings? Kim's family?

Gradually, I was able to piece it together. The caller was our close friend from Orlando, my former colleague at WESH Lisa Rayam. We knew she and Lee Norris had gone to Jamaica to celebrate the two-year anniversary of their wedding, that moving ceremony in which they serenaded one another. Between sobs, Lisa was saying something about some craftsmen she and

Lee Norris had met on the beach. I heard the words "break-in." And "gone." As in, "Lee Norris is gone."

Gone. Murdered.

The story started to become clear. How Lisa and Lee Norris had encountered some local craftsmen selling wood carvings on the beach at Runaway Bay, the resort community where they'd rented a villa. How they didn't buy anything from the vendors, but that didn't stop Lee Norris from giving them some money anyway. That's the kind of guy Lee Norris was: generous, kind. How, that night, they were awakened by sounds of someone breaking into their villa. How they jumped out of bed and tried to hold the bedroom door closed while a man or men fought to push it open. How, in the struggle, as the door pushed open, Lisa recognized one of the local craftsmen from the beach before getting hit in the head. How she didn't even remember the gunshot that had murdered her husband.

"Take all the time you need." That's what my bosses at ESPN said the next morning. It would be the first in a long series: Throughout my time at the Worldwide Leader, the executives who ran the place defied the cold, heartless corporate stereotype. Time and again, they led with their heart.

So, the next morning, Kim and I boarded a flight for Miami, where we met up with Lee Norris's two brothers, and on we all went to Jamaica. We went straight to the hospital, which felt third-rate and dirty. Lee Norris's body hadn't even been cleaned up yet. Lisa was adamant that she wasn't leaving Jamaica without her husband's body, but the police weren't releasing it. The Jamaican tourist board put all of us up at a luxury hotel, and the countdown started as we all had to wait for the bureaucracy to move. Jamaica is totally laid-back, which is fine if you're having a relaxing vacation and don't run into any problems. But when the stakes are high and you need action, the wheels of justice are frustratingly slow. Kim and I weren't going to let Lisa go through this alone, and my bosses agreed: "Stay there," they all but demanded of me.

We were in Jamaica for over a week. Even though Lisa had her own room at the hotel, she stayed in ours the first four nights. On Saturday morning we heard Lisa start singing. Her voice had always been on loan from God, and singing was always something she and Lee Norris shared in a very deep way. The day she started singing she said to us, "I think I want to spend some quiet time alone," and she went to her room.

So much of our time had been spent worrying about Lisa that Kim and I hadn't had time to grieve. We both broke down. So much emotion had built up that the floodgates just swung open. We made love.

Now, there's a backstory here. When Kim and I had first gotten married, the doctors discovered she had trouble conceiving. She had surgery, and her doctor told us that if we were planning on having children, we'd better hurry up and get on it. In late '93, we started trying—and trying and trying. It was actually kind of funny. Since Kim was a flight attendant, and I was married to her, I could fly for free. She'd call when the opportunity was ripe, and I'd hop on a plane to do my husbandly duty. One time she was in Missoula, Montana, when I got the call: "I'm ovulating." Nine hours later, I was in Montana, doing "calisthenics" with the wife. Despite these efforts, we still had no luck getting pregnant.

Shortly after our time in Jamaica with Lisa, though, we got word: We were expecting. We sat down with a calendar and did the math and figured out that we had conceived on that Saturday when Lisa felt strong enough to stay in her own room.

We called Lisa and told her God had taken a life—and God had given a life. We told her that Lee Norris was our child's guardian angel. I'm not a Bible-thumper, but I am a Christian and I do pray and I do believe His will works mysteriously. Need proof? Taelor was born on February 20, 1995. It was Lee Norris's birthday. I told you: life. What a trip, man.

LET'S KEEP IT REAL. Like most dads who are jocks, I kinda wanted a son. While Kim was pregnant, I wanted to know our baby's sex. Friends weighed in: Keep the surprise factor, some advised. There's no right answer. The right answer is you do what you want to do.

And I wanted to know. I felt like I *needed* to know, because I wanted to know who I was talking to while I bonded with my child throughout the pregnancy. I wanted to know if I'd be saying "Hey, baby girl" or "Hey, big boy." I was gonna talk to that belly—and saying "Hey, baby" struck me as plain stupid.

After the doctor told us it was a girl, I remember driving back from his office that day and thinking, *This is the best thing in the world. I'm gonna have a baby girl.* All that stuff about having a son was instantly gone; once I knew, I was all in.

The day Taelor was first put in my arms I was a changed man. Every dad is biased, of course, but c'mon: She was the most beautiful baby I'd ever seen. Five pounds, eight ounces, with a full head of hair. Her eyes were closed and she was blowing bubbles.

There are probably a million ways to describe what it's like to have a kid. Every one of them rings true. Here's mine: When that baby is put into your arms, she is instantaneously set apart from everyone else in your life, even your significant other. When you first meet your child, she becomes the only person—ever—with whom you are already deeply, deeply in love. And the love does nothing but grow from there.

I was a fanatical father. It bothered me that I couldn't produce milk. I so wanted to be a part of that. I told my wife, as if to compensate, "I'm changing every diaper when I'm home. I'm here, I'm changing the diaper."

Kim would fly for work on my off days. If Kim was gone for a couple of days and I had the same days off work, Taelor and I would hit the road. Sometimes we'd fly to North Carolina to see my folks, or we'd visit Kim, or we'd go hang out with my boy Fred, who was now in Florida. I can't tell you how much I loved traveling with Taelor. It was not the normal thing for a man to do. One time, I was in a stall in the ESPN bathroom when a couple of colleagues walked in—to this day, I don't know who they were. One said, "Wife's going out of town this weekend, leaving our two-year-old with me; what am I going to do?"

"Yeah, my wife did that to me once," the other dude said. "I didn't know what to do all weekend."

I was sitting there on the toilet thinking, *What is wrong with you guys? You can't stay with your own kid?* I wanted to smack them.

I was proud to travel with my kid. I had it down to a science. I wasn't fumbling around like some amateur. I packed a bag; I had the carrier; I'd take the bottles out on the plane and ask the attendant to put them on ice for the flight. It was like clockwork.

Still, people had a hard time wrapping their heads around the sight of the two of us, and it ticked me off. Whether we were in the security line at the airport, boarding a plane, or checking into a hotel, someone would inevitably say: "Oh, look. Mr. Mom." People were trying to be nice—complimentary, even. But I hated that. I'm not Mr. Mom—I'm Dad. Is Mom ever *Mrs. Dad*?

Or how about this one: "Oh, that's so sweet. Dad's babysitting." Seriously? Babysitters get paid. I'm no babysitter. I'm Dad. That sense of surprise, that inability to process the fact of a dad who was as conscientious as a mom—it's a sad commentary on what our culture expects from fathers.

Kim was out of town for my first Father's Day in June 1995. I got Taelor up and made her breakfast, and then we went to a horse pasture a few blocks from our house. I held her real close to the fence as the horses sidled up and we'd talk to them. And we'd talk to each other: one thing I never did with Taelor or Sydni was speak to them in singsong baby talk. I think that's why both were so conversational early on and grew up to be well-read and social. I always talked to them like they were adults. That day—even though Taelor was only five months old—I told her all about everyone in her family, even her great-grandfather, my mom's dad.

"He died back in 1941," I said. "He was murdered. He went to get milk for his kids, who were in the bathtub. He walked down the street and got mugged and shot."

That's how I talked to her—a real adult conversation, before she could even talk back. So I wasn't surprised when she became talkative. I remember sitting in a Cincinnati restaurant when Taelor was eighteen months old, and Kim and I counted how many words our baby girl knew: 153. One time, when she was about three, we were in a Barnes & Noble bookstore and I asked the lady who worked there for a certain book for Taelor. "Oh, those books are for kids nine or ten years old," she said. "Your girl is too young for it."

Oh, yeah? Today, I might shrug and say, "No, really, she can read that book." Back then, it was a challenge. "Grab one," I barked to the unsuspecting clerk. "Get me a book."

The book in front of her, Taelor just started reading. Clutch. I leaned back, crossed my arms, and glared at the clerk. Like, really, lady?

Suddenly, I was no longer in much of a hurry to hang with my boys. Taelor was my best buddy. Before I'd leave for work in the morning, I'd head to Taelor's room. "Hey," Kim would call after me, "don't wake her up."

"I won't," I'd say. "Just gonna see if she's up. If she is, I'll just say good-bye."

Well, so much for that. I'd walk into the room and she'd be sound asleep. "Pssst, Taelor, baby girl, wake up," I'd whisper, nudging her. I couldn't help myself. If I was going to spend the next twelve to eighteen hours at work, I needed a fix. I'd pick her up and bring her downstairs, where Kim would greet us with a disbelieving look.

"Look who was up," I'd say. "I figured I'd bring her down and spend some time with her."

When Taelor was two, we had friends over for New Year's Eve. As we got closer to midnight, I snuck away and headed upstairs. She was up—though, honestly, I would have woken her up. I started to rock her in the rocking chair we had in her bedroom. As I rocked her, the emotion of the moment hit me. Another year was about to end, and my baby girl was already two; I started to feel the passage of time. I started to feel overwhelmingly blessed to have this little life in mine. I'd always felt things deeply, and now it was all too much. The tears started streaming down my cheeks.

Taelor raised her head, looking at me, frowning slightly. "Daddy, are you crying?"

I smiled. "Yeah, Daddy's crying," I said, sniffling.

She got up, and I bent down to her. She touched my cheek. "Are those tears of joy, Daddy?"

"Yeah, baby girl," I said. "Those are tears of joy."

AFTER A COUPLE OF YEARS, *SportsNight* was becoming less focused on rock climbing and surfing. More and more, we were giving the same scores and highlights as *SportsCenter*. It didn't make sense to have both. Once *SportsNight* went away in 1995, my colleagues all made the jump to prime-time *SportsCenter*. Suzy. Kenny Mayne. Bill Pidto.

All but me. Granted, I already had a show: I was doing *NBA2Nite*, which I liked just fine. But not getting the call for *SportsCenter* gnawed at me. Oftentimes, we want the shiniest thing and we're going to huff and puff about it till we get it. I went to my bosses and let them know what I wanted. The word kept coming back: "Your time will come."

I felt like I was being patted on the head, but what could I do?

I kept telling myself that, ultimately, I could only control what I could control. That, while I was watching Suzy, Kenny, and Bill anchor our network's flagship show—and I was legitimately happy for them—I needed to kick butt on *NBA2Nite*. The rest would take care of itself.

Why was I the last of the *SportsNight* crew to graduate to *SportsCenter*? Beats me. Questions of "why" always perplex me. Even today, Kristin will ask me, "Why do you think so-and-so said that?" and my response is always the same: I don't know, so why waste the time and energy trying to figure it out? What's important is what we *know*. And, back then, I knew I had to deal with not being called up to *SportsCenter*, and that it was up to me to perform in a way that would make it impossible to be overlooked again.

My boys would wonder if it had to do with race. I thought that was too easy an out. I didn't see myself as a victim—particularly when there's *real* discrimination out there. If forced to speculate, I'd say I wouldn't be surprised if there *were* doubts about me among the network's higher-ups—but that they wouldn't be based on how different I looked. I bet it was more about how I acted. I wouldn't be surprised if there was a feeling that I was little more than a catchphrase guy. A young dude with an entertaining shtick.

I sensed that that perception changed one night in the summer of 1996 when Rece Davis and I were cohosting the two a.m. *SportsCenter*. The Centenniel Olympic Park in Atlanta had just been bombed. Our sleepy studio burst into action. The script was ripped from the teleprompter. This was live TV and there'd be no net. We were on the air till ten a.m., winging it. That night, more than anything else, changed how I was looked at by the bigwigs in Bristol and New York.

They might have seen me as some excitable jock, but the fact is I was a veteran of live TV news. Remember, I'd been a local news reporter. And I'd always been a fan of Peter Jennings. I'd watch how, on big stories, he projected a sense of calm and comfort. Most viewers would watch him to get the information he was putting out there. I'd watch him to try to figure out how he did what he did and what made him so good at it.

I knew it was hard because when a big story breaks your natural tendency is to be amped up—the adrenaline starts flowing. I concentrated on slowing down, even as things were firing at me. It's a tricky balancing act: You want to project an air of serene authority, but you also want to have energy in your voice. And you have to pull off that careful balance while producers are shrieking in your ear all the while.

Rece would be questioning the chief medical examiner of Atlanta–Fulton County Stadium, who was on the satellite, while the producer in my ear was telling us that, in one minute, they'd kick it to me to interview the head of security for the International Olympic Committee. No script and no time to prepare. That's when you think of your folks back home or your boys and you wonder: What would *they* want to know right now? So I'd ask about whether there had been any elevated threat levels leading up to this, if there were any suspects. I'd keep the queries coming—how robust had the security been compared to past Games?—until that voice in my ear, with no warning, would shout, "Gotta go, gotta go!" Then it's time to wrap up the interview in a way that looks planned before Rece and I engage in some respectful byplay—some interaction that humanizes us and allows the viewer to pause and react for him- or herself.

ESPN and CNN were the first on the air to report the bombing, but the rush to be first means nothing if what you're producing isn't top quality. And we aced it that night. That was no accident. ESPN in the early to mid-nineties was setting a high bar for smart coverage of big news stories, and that came straight from the top. When highly respected John Walsh, who had been an editor at both *Rolling Stone* and the *Washington Post* and founding editor of *Inside Sports* magazine, joined the network in the late eighties as vice president and executive editor, he brought with him hard-news credibility. He started to build a journalistic culture.

Walsh is a fascinating character. His friends through the years have included Hunter S. Thompson and Bill Murray. He preached the importance of hard, unbiased news reporting at a sports network—something of an oxymoron at the time. The direct result of Walsh's influence would soon be found in ESPN's leading coverage of the O. J. Simpson case and on that night in 1996, when Rece and I spent six hours on the air reporting the Olympic bombing.

After that night, I received personalized notes from many ESPN executives, all praising the job I'd done. I'd shown the ability to think on my feet and ask insightful questions. I wasn't just some excitable kid. Almost right away, my time did indeed come. I got my shot anchoring *SportsCenter*. In 2014, just before we unveiled our new state-of-the-art *SportsCenter* set, I was asked to look back at my initial broadcast for a promotional piece called "First Show. First Set."

There I was, alongside Craig Kilborn, on that pale *SportsCenter* set. I had a thick dark mustache, and I wore my hair in a type of baby high-top fade, which was all the rage among young black men at the time: short on the sides, long on top. But the thing that really captured my eye was the big, boxy tan suit. "This is back in the day," I said, "when suits were boxy, with big shoulders. Now everything is Euro, slim-fit. Back in the day, big and baggy was cool. There are still some brothers who will wear suits like that. Not a lot of brothers." Here I paused, about to level a loving shot to one of my whitest colleagues: "Some brothers. And Barry Melrose."

That's what I saw, looking back at that clip from September 1996: a young black man rocking the style of the day. But I also saw something else, something harder for the naked eye to make out. I saw a dude who had been given the freedom to let his voice fly.

CHAPTER SIX

DROPPIN' KNOWLEDGE

Remember when Iron Mike Tyson burst onto the scene in the eighties? He'd intimidate his opponent in the pre-fight stare-down. It would be over before the first punch. Rappers got it—here was a dude whose in-your-face attitude came straight outta their lyrics. LL Cool J gave Iron Mike props: *"I'm Mike Tyson, icin', I'm a soldier at war/Makin' sure you don't try to battle me no more."* Big Daddy Kane weighed in: *"My sharp tongue is like a license/I strike like Mike Tyson."* There were other ballers, too, who seemed ripped from the pages of *The Source* magazine. Public Enemy singled out a beefy power forward: *"Throw down like Barkley!"* Chuck D shouted.

But by the mid-nineties, right around the time I started anchoring *SportsCenter,* something changed. Rappers weren't just shouting out to athletes. Now rappers and sports stars were becoming one. Interchangeable. That's because a generation of athletes who had grown up on hip-hop came onto the scene—and they looked and acted different from those who had come before.

I was there in Orlando when Shaq started rhyming with Fu-Schnickens. Around the same time, Michigan's Fab Five, led by Chris Webber and Jalen Rose, with their shaved heads and baggy shorts, were bringing urban style into the mainstream. Then

Allen Iverson, with his cornrows, his tats, and his "posse" of rapping friends burst into the NBA, and a new era had dawned. The hip-hop athlete was born.

Pretty soon, a whole lot of black athletes were wearing the hip-hop uniform: the droopy pants, the Enyce and Ecko gear, the braids and tats. As for the music, many followed Shaq's lead and dropped some science of their own: Roy Jones Jr. and "Prime Time" Deion Sanders both tried their hands at the rap game. Later, so many would do the same—including Kobe and A.I.— that it had a name: They were "rapletes."

What was going on? Suddenly hip-hop's influence was everywhere in sports, because hip-hop had become the driving force of youth culture. It went beyond race; after all, something like 70 percent of all rap music back then was bought by white kids in the suburbs. And it was about more than the music; if you were young and interested in pop culture, hip-hop influenced how you spoke and carried yourself.

By the time I got to *SportsCenter*, the impact of hip-hop was everywhere . . . except in the sports broadcast booth. My industry seemed black-and-white in the Technicolor hip-hop world, with our well-coiffed, deep-voiced anchors and their perfect diction. All that passion in our sports and music? It wasn't often found in the media reporting of the game.

GQ magazine called me the "hip-hop Howard Cosell"; I guess I was being held up as representative of this new generation. I say "I guess" because this is me, now, looking back. I thought about none of this back in the day. You think I was sitting around, saying to myself, "Self, you gotta represent hip-hop nation on *SportsCenter* tonight?" Man, I was busy high-fiving my boys after watching Mike come back from his baseball sabbatical by dropping a double nickel on the Knicks. Who had time to think about what it all meant?

But now I think that's partly why what I was doing on-air caught on. Because it wasn't calculated. I was just being myself, writing and talking about sports the way I would with Stephen or Fred or any one of my boys. And that came through. Listen to rap music back then; hip-hop was all about authenticity. If someone "kept it real"—that was the highest of compliments. Viewers are smart; they can tell who is genuine and who is running game.

Within a couple of years, I was making a cameo in the rapper Luke's "Raise the Roof" video. Luke was a legend; back in the day, he and his boys in the 2 Live Crew were charged by Florida authorities with breaking obscenity laws in their music. Their album *As Nasty As They Wanna Be* came out in 1989, and their lyrics *were* pretty far out there. I was more of a Luther Vandross and old-school rap kind of guy. I was partial to the inoffensive Sugarhill Gang. But I had much respect for how Luke handled being public enemy number one. When the Florida governor banned his music and the sheriff arrested him, Luke said elected leaders should focus on ending poverty instead of his music. Made sense to me. Ultimately, the courts vindicated him.

Luke reached out and said he had a part for me as the "announcer" at a house party. Whoa, hold on, I said. I told him it sounded cool, but—knowing his history for pushing the envelope—ESPN would have to sign off before I said yes. I couldn't do anything that wasn't straight with the network's image. Turned out, there was nothing to worry about. It was a fun party video—the song ended up being Luke's biggest hit. It began with me dressed all in black looking into the camera, the house party raging behind me, and saying: "Hey, what's going on there. Stuart Scott for WLUK-TV." Then Luke, with help from others—including Ice Cube and Puff Daddy in cameos of their own—introduced America to the Raise the Roof dance craze, in which, palms up, you thrust your arms skyward. Periodically, the camera would swing back to me: "Look, it's not that difficult," I said, demonstrating the move. "You just get up, take one hand, the other hand, and just . . . raise the roof!" At one point, I'm watching the action and turn to the camera: "Off da heezy!" I exclaim. That's black, y'all, for "This is a wild time."

It was cool because what I was doing in the video wasn't that different from what I was bringing to *SportsCenter*: I was hosting a party. Every night, I was expressing myself, celebrating sports the way I did while I was growing up. I think that attitude—*This is sports, man; let's have fun with it*—resonated with viewers, especially younger ones.

The catchphrases helped people take notice, no question. People still want to talk to me about them. Funny thing is, catchphrases are not nearly as big a deal to us on-air guys as they are to the audience. It's not like we sit around and put in time trying to come up with them. They just tend to happen. I might think of something, or be reminded of something, and think, *Hey, I could use that.* And a catchphrase is born.

On-air catchphrases at ESPN became a thing. Anchors had the freedom to riff—and that set us apart from how sports had always been reported. The way we did it, we were saying to the viewer: Yo, man, we don't take ourselves too seriously here. And if you tune in, you might just chuckle to yourself over a clever pop-culture reference or a parody of a hard-to-pronounce name. And who doesn't need a good laugh now and again?

It started with Chris Berman, of course: "He . . . could . . . go . . . all . . . the . . . way!" or "Marshall, Marshall, Marshall!" Craig Kilborn: "Don't fake the funk on a nasty dunk." Dan Patrick: "He's listed as day-to-day, but aren't we all?" Robin Roberts: "Get down with your bad self!" Steve Levy: "It's the NBA, and everybody makes a run." Scott Van Pelt: "Slappa!" John Buccigross: "Winner, winner, chicken dinner."

You weren't hearing that kind of voice anywhere else in the sports world. In fact, you weren't getting *any* pop-culture references anywhere else—because sports had always been covered like it was its own private world, cut off from everyday life.

REMEMBER, THE ROOTS OF *Boo-yah!* were back in Winston-Salem, when Fred's neighbor, Mr. G, the oldhead who made bamboo chairs, used it once to describe how loud the previous night's thunder had been. From then on, we'd say it when someone brought a different kind of thunder on the field or court. A slam dunk in your face? *Boo-yah!* A blindside flattening of the QB? *Boo-yah!*

Someone once told me I got "cool as the other side of the pillow" from a movie, but that's not the case. Back when I was in Florence, South Carolina, barely staying afloat on all of two hundred bucks a week and trying to soak up as much knowledge as I could at my first job in TV, I was so poor, I had no air-conditioning in my apartment. Guess how I used to cool off at night? I'd flip that pillow to the cool side and get a momentary rush. I started working it into my scripts on the air. It was a way to have some voice, to say something in an original way.

One day, we were watching some baller light it up in a game somewhere when my former brother-in-law said, "Call that dude butter 'cause he's on a roll." I cracked up and took ownership of it and can now offer props to Calvin, my former bro-in-law.

A lot of my catchphrases came from my life as an African-American—and they were things other black people could relate to. "That's so good, make you want to sop it up with a biscuit," I'd say. I'd look for ways to play off current pop-culture happenings, like when Michael would go off from downtown: "Michael, Michael, Michael, can't you see, sometimes your threes just hypnotize me," I said, sampling Biggie Smalls. Sometimes I'd be speaking straight to the African-American viewer: "Lawd, he done made his kinfolk proud: Pookie 'n' dem, Big Mama 'n' dem . . ." or "He's got more flavor than Kool-Aid and cocoa." One of my home-run calls came from Sunday morning, in my best Southern Baptist preacher voice: "And the Lawd said you got to rise up, we gonna open the doors of the *chutch*"—not "church" but "*chutch*." Those ones are just for us, okay? If you grew up black and in the South, you knew what I was talking about. You had an Uncle Pookie and Big Mama at your barbecues, your fridge was always stocked with Kool-Aid or Hi-C, and the voice of the preacher man would always be renting space in your head.

I guess I didn't realize how much all of it was resonating out there until 1999, when *Saturday Night Live* aired a parody of me—and my catchphrases. It was eye-opening for me. *Wow, I remember thinking, I guess I am this thing called a "celebrity."*

The skit starred Tim Meadows as me and Ray Romano as new, overenthused anchor Chet Harper on the set of *SportsCenter.* "Shaq-Daddy with 37 points—he sends an invitation to the Finals party, and it says 'B.Y.O.B.': 'Bring your own *Boo-yah!*'" Tim Meadows, er, I said over footage of Shaq throwing down.

Then it was the newcomer's turn, and he took things further into the weird than I'd ever go. "Latest talk is that David Robinson is over the hill," Romano's Harper said, over clips of the Spurs. "But in my book, you gotta get to White Castle before the weirdos show up! Tonight at the Alamodome, he gets happy-go-Jackie on the big white guy like a donkey eating a waffle! Sweet sassy molassey! Get out the checkbook and pay Grandma for the rubdown as the Spurs beat the Heat, 86–79!"

Harper's catchphrases grew increasingly out-there: "John Stockton says, 'Hey, look at me, I'm a little teapot; I'll run right up your dress'"; a hockey goalie says, "Hey, try not to shoot that puck up my pooper!"; a goal-scorer "celebrates like a slave who made it to the North!"

It was funny and brilliant. It was a parody of me, but, in the sketch, my character was actually the *straight* man. Ray Romano's character extended what I do to the hilariously absurd. More than a decade later, I'd run into Romano at Michael Jordan's golf tournament. I'd become a fan of his TNT show, *Men of a Certain Age,* the story of three best friends in their late forties dealing with the onset of middle age, also starring Andre Braugher and Scott Bakula. And Romano is part of the ensemble cast of *Parenthood,* another of my favorite shows.

So I was psyched to meet him. Before I could find him, he found me—to tell me his son was a fan of *mine*. "Before I came here, he asked, 'Is Stuart Scott going to be there?'" he said.

Then he tripped me out. He started apologizing for the *SNL* skit. "You know, I didn't write that thing—" he said.

"You kidding, man?" I said. "That put me on the map. I loved it!"

Clearly, *SNL* had tapped into something. The catchphrases were popular, but they weren't my focus. Writing great copy was the priority. I'd spend hours writing each night's show—only you had to write in such a way that it looked like you didn't spend *any* time writing it. I knew that as a loud, young, African-American anchor my work was going to be put under a microscope. That's when I determined that, alongside the catchphrases, nods to urban life, and pop-culture references, I needed to give you *more* hard-core sports information than anyone else. I got me a notebook and kept running tallies of which among us on-air personalities gave out the most statistics. It was usually me. My own personal edict became "I'm going to tell you *more*": more points, more rebounds, more batting averages, more home runs, more touchdown passes. I knew I was going to be judged differently, so I wanted cold, hard data to show that I was providing more information than anyone else doing this job.

There are great researchers at ESPN, and I wouldn't leave them poor boys alone. I'd call them up and be, like, "How many times did A.I. score 40 this year? Is that more or less than Jordan?" Ten minutes later, I'd ring back: "Yo, man, Steve Young—how does he compare with Elway on fourth-quarter comebacks?"

Very few people pay attention to good writing on TV broadcasts, but it's one thing that sets ESPN apart. I'm not saying I'm the best writer in Bristol, but even in my earliest days at the Worldwide Leader I knew I could write with anybody on that campus. Now, I'm not talking about writing the King's English, about using ten-karat words to show off how smart you are. I'm talking about writing that doesn't sound like writing. I'm talking about writing that sounds like you're sitting right there in the viewer's man cave, having a conversation.

I spend hours writing my intros—the pieces that set up the highlights, where anchors are looking directly into the camera. That's when we have the most freedom to be creative. Last year, for example, when the lowly Philadelphia 76ers visited the great San Antonio Spurs, I wrote a "two neighborhoods, two teams" setup that talked about how they were teams from the opposite sides of town. In talking about the Spurs, I was dressed in an immaculate suit; when I got to the Sixers—thanks to great editing— my suit became torn and disheveled and I looked like I was down and out on the street. It was a creative, dramatic way to get across the theme of that night's game: two franchises going in two very different directions.

But even during the highlights, *SportsCenter* anchors are not satisfied doing the same-old, same-old scores and highlights. Here's a snippet of me doing a highlight of a touchdown pass and then a sack in a game between the New York Giants and the Jacksonville Jaguars: "*The very next play, Collins gets silly-nutty with Ron Dixon—8 yards. Dixon—talk about nibboo!—Baryshnikov!— oh! Just getting both feet in—14–zip G-Men. Third quarter, 17–nothing Giants—uh-oh—Michael Strahan about to put the beat-down clock down on Mark Brunell. Yeah, dawg—we know that.*"

This is something I always stress to broadcast students: It may not read or sound like it, but as many hours of thought and re-writing go into my *SportsCenter* scripts as, say, Peter Jennings would put into his for *World News Tonight*.

What I do might not appear to be journalism, but it is. Some-times other journalists don't even get that. Early on, there were detractors of mine who would say I was buddies with athletes and that you can't be a good journalist if that's the case. Sports radio talker Mike Francesa once said that I'll "slap hands with [a player] or have some little cute response with him or something that almost in some way hints at friendship as much as I'm here to cover you."

Now, what Mike Francesa thinks of me is none of my busi-ness. I don't know how I developed it, but even in my early thir-ties, I had an "I don't care" attitude when I heard stuff like that. Because I knew what the criticism was really about. Yes, I am friends with some athletes. The people I admire and respect who are athletes are people I'd admire and respect if they *weren't* athletes.

But I think a couple of other things were going on. One was that the athletes I covered were of my generation; they'd been tuning in to *SportsCenter* for fifteen years, and maybe now they were finally hearing someone speak like them. It stands to reason they'd be more open and comfortable with me, that we'd have more of a connection.

But I also think the criticism I got early on really came from not getting our role as journalists. You've heard me say it before: I'm interested in explaining, not judging. And athletes get when they talk to me that I'm not playing "gotcha." The rapport I have with athletes comes not from slapping hands with them but from having played sports. It helps to have competed at some level— not because I know what it feels like to catch a touchdown pass but because I know what it feels like to *drop* it. If I can ask a question that gets across that I get it, that I know what you're going through, the answer coming back is going to be more open and interesting.

That's what happened last year, after Miami's only win of the NBA Finals against the Spurs. At the end of the game, LeBron had driven and dished to Chris Bosh for a big shot. When I got Bosh after the game, I could have just asked the pro forma "What were you thinking when you hit that clutch shot?" Guys are so used to that question, they tend to pull out a tried-and-true cliché.

I decided to ask two questions. The first: "We all know that athletes see plays before they actually happen. When did you see that play happen?"

"First, after we called it," responded Bosh, who is a really thoughtful guy. "But then when I saw LeBron driving and he drew two guys, I knew it was coming to me."

Then I asked: "What were you thinking when you let it fly?"

"Nothing," Bosh said. "I know a lot of guys say, 'I was thinking this' or 'I was thinking that.' I wasn't thinking anything. I just let it fly."

I love that exchange, because it was simple and true. The first question got at, from an athlete's perspective, how things really happen out there. I've talked to LeBron and others about this: All say there are times when the game slows down for them and they know what's going to happen before it actually does. That enabled the second question—and I love Bosh's answer because it's so true. Shots go in *because* you were able to shut down the distracting thoughts of your own mind. To me, that's journalism that serves the viewer's understanding of the game.

There was only one time that an athlete got on me for something I said about him on the air. Remember big Oliver Miller of the Phoenix Suns? We played a clip of him dribbling out on a fast break and dunking. I said, "Look at Big O—he can eat all them Twinkies and still get up!"

Four months later, I saw him in the locker room and he wasn't happy. "Man, you were talking smack about me!"

"What'd I say?" I asked, even though I thought I knew.

"I don't know, but you were talking 'bout me," he said.

"I remember what I said, man. I said you can eat all them Twinkies and still get up. I wasn't busting on you for being a big dude, I was saying you're a big dude and you can still throw it down! Man, your nickname is the Big O."

He kind of smiled and we hugged it out. There's only one other confrontation I can remember. Brian Williams was drafted out of Arizona by the Magic when I was in Orlando. (He later changed his name to Bison Dele and died mysteriously at sea, presumably killed by his brother.) One day in Orlando's locker room back then, he walked over to me and said, "Why'd you give my address out?"

I didn't know what he was talking about. He was towering over me. "I didn't give your address out," I said. "What are you talking about?"

He grabbed me. "Why'd you give my address out?" he said, harder now.

I just reacted. "Take your freakin' hands off me," I said through gritted teeth, staring up about eleven inches.

I grabbed his wrists and said it again. He turned and walked away. I never did find out what in the world he was talking about.

See, I think it's pretty good that I can think of only two times when an athlete has been ticked off at me—and one wasn't even for anything I actually did. That's because I don't think my role is to be antagonistic. My role is to help the viewer get who these guys are, and to understand the game better.

In 1999, just before announcing that Vince Carter—Tar Heel!—was the runaway Rookie of the Year, I broke down a dunk by him that everyone had been calling a 360-degree throw-down. Only it wasn't. "I gotta drop some knowledge," I said, while footage of Vince's slam played on the screen behind me. "Vince Carter's late-season 360 dunk was not *really* a 360. Let me show you." At this, we played a clip of a recent Kobe 360. "Most guys do a true 360—they start to their right, complete the circle, slam it."

Now we played Vince's. "Vince basically did, like, a 450—he started the other way, went all the way *around* before ripping the rim."

It was a little thing, and it wasn't going to win any awards. No broadcast journalism professor was going to show it to his or her class. But it was helping the viewer see something in a new way. It was me, doing what I saw as my role. Droppin' knowledge.

WE ALL KNOW from sports how hard it is to have staying power. Teams that look like they can become dynasties get complacent or unlucky—or some combination of both. Before you know it, they go from champion back to also-ran. So how did ESPN do it? It was a sports network run out of a couple of beat-up trailers in barren Bristol, Connecticut, in the 1970s. Today, the same turf that housed those trailers is now home to a 123-acre campus with twenty buildings and a bottom line that other networks covet. It's one of the nation's premier brands—transcending sports. How did it happen? What's the secret to ESPN's success?

I'm no expert when it comes to business, but I think I know enough about the culture of ESPN to know the answer. It can be summed up in one word: vision. It's something that is in short supply in the business world. But not at ESPN.

Guys like former president George Bodenheimer, current president John Skipper, and John Walsh have it in spades. They're the smartest guys I know. And they're never willing to let the brand rest on its laurels—the culture they've established is one that always encourages trying new things.

I've never met people who think more about what's next than these dudes. Take the network's current $5.6 billion deal with Major League Baseball. Yes, it gives us the rights to televise regular-season and playoff games until 2021, along with all high-light, international, and radio rights. But it did something else, because Skipper knew where the future was heading: It gave ESPN the right to stream all that content through its mobile apps. It should come as no surprise that, now, more than 70 percent of all content consumed on mobile apps comes courtesy of ESPN. It's because guys like Skipper were always thinking about the new when it came to "new media." A tall Southern transplant who still speaks with a drawl, Skipper's first job was at *Rolling Stone* magazine—just like Walsh. These guys weren't business school numbers-crunchers. They were passionate about the product.

That's what has set ESPN apart since I joined the team. The guys in charge value creativity and diversity in radical ways.

We were encouraged to be creative in the moment, even while on live TV. If we were having fun on the set, the thinking went, the viewer will have fun watching us. Remember that time 50 Cent threw out the first pitch at a Pirates–Mets game and the ball went at least a hundred feet wide of home plate? We couldn't stop showing it. I was, like, "Dude, don't you practice? That's not even close."

The same night, the USA soccer team played Azerbaijan in a World Cup warm-up match. The World Cup would be starting in fifteen days. For some reason, I was assuming the team must have already left the States—and that this game was in Azerbaijan. I knew that our Bob Ley would be covering the World Cup, so I figured he was there with them. I threw it to him with the intro: "Let's go to Bob Ley, in Azerbaijan with Team USA."

While Bob was doing his stand-up, the producer in my ear clued me in to a pretty big oversight on my part. When the red light in front of me came back on, I decided on the spot to come clean.

"Thanks, Bob," I said. "As you can see, Bob is not in Azerbaijan. Bob is not even in San Francisco tonight, where the match is actually being played. If you walk out right behind me, outside our studio door, hang a right, Bob Ley is right down that hall."

Now, that was funny. But what was funnier was a viewer's tweet to me, which we instantly put on screen and closed the show with: "What do you and 50 Cent have in common? You both tossed to Azerbaijan instead of sixty feet away."

In that case, as in so many others, we made the viewer a part of the fun. That mind-set comes from the top. I've always had the freedom to think up new ways to get across the same old information. For me, those ways often reflected the African-American experience—which gets to the diversity ingredient of Skipper's secret sauce.

Take, for example, my spoken-word *SportsCenter* segments. Instead of delivering the typical scores and highlights, I've come out on set to a live mic and, behind some old-school jazz, laid down some poetry jam. There was the Kentucky–Florida basketball game:

> *Kentucky's Terrence Jones drives*
> *To his surprise*
> *The shot won't go and Florida starts to run*
> *In b-ball it's called transition*
> *Of your own volition*
> *Step on the gas pedal*
> *Heavy metal*
> *Fire under the kettle*
> *Whatever you want to call it*
> *Call it a Patric Young dunk*
> *Kid brought the funk . . .*
> *Gators down two*
> *But who knew?*

Kentucky's freshman big man could be this clean
Anthony Davis sets the screen
Steps back beyond the line
Tickles the twine
From three.

Name one place where an anchor wouldn't be laughed off the set if he suggested rapping old-school over scores and highlights. In early 2014, I gave Steph Curry the *SportsCenter* poetry-jam treatment:

Part of a 30–5 Warriors run
Steph wasn't done
Shooting from distance not working so much
Young fella drives, twists
Serious touch.

Again, writing. It doesn't take as long as you might think to write one of these. You have to see the video first and then write to it—but then it's all a matter of flow. Rhyming for spoken word is made easier because you can speed up or slow down your pace to make the rhyme. My favorite spoken-word segment came a few years ago, when I paid tribute to Mike in "Best Ever" on his fiftieth birthday:

Brotha, I was sold when he won six NBA rings
But the thing
That makes Best Ever sing
Not scoring titles and MVPs

The double nickel that he sliced the Knicks at their knees
The 63 he put on Bird
Larry Legend saying "Please!
Is that God?"
Isn't it odd
That Best Ever is not about numbers
But whatever he made you feel
Just watching
Shock, then awe
Then amazing that drops your jaw
Might be pride or scorn
Depending on whether you were born
A Bulls, Knicks, or Celtics fan
Man, he's even better than Best Ever
In a career he has weathered every storm
Paved the way for athletes to say "I am an icon"
A brand
Over my likeness I stand
On this day we stand tall, too
Honoring you
Michael Jordan
Best Ever.
Happy birthday, black cat. Spoken word.

Twitter blows up when I break out a spoken-word jam. Not everybody likes it, though most do. But here's what Bodenheimer, Skipper, and Walsh all knew: It's *okay* if not everybody likes it. If you try to please *everybody* you succeed in just being bland most of the time.

That was part of my argument last year, when one pro-ducer objected to one of my most recent catchphrases. When, say, Yasiel Puig went yard against Justin Verlander, I played off a popular Kendrick Lamar song and said, "Puig to Verlander: Pitch, don't kill my vibe!"

Every time I used the line, the Twitter audience loved it. But one producer was offended—not at what I'd said, but at Lamar's original lyric, which substituted a *B* for the *P* in pitch.

"Look, man," I told the dude. "This is what we do. We bor-row from culture and create things out of it that have to do with sports."

"But it uses the word 'bitch,'" he said.

"But it's *'pitch,'*" I said. "I'm taking a Kendrick Lamar title and making it baseball-centric. You gotta understand, man, I've got two daughters at home so I'm aware of the sensitivity we need to show here." What I was doing was no different from what another anchor used to do, borrowing from that viral Dave Chappelle skit where Chappelle and Wayne Brady are cruising the 'hood, acting all gangsta, and Brady, the most unthreatening black man, keeps saying, "Is Wayne Brady going to have to choke a bitch?" Well, anytime we showed highlights of tennis great Novak Djokovic, my colleague used to say, "Is Novak going to have to Djokovic?" The only difference is that none of the producers *got* that reference.

I kept using the phrase, after the producer and I had a high-minded conversation about it that I appreciated. But the key take-away for me is that a show producer raised the objection—not one of the executives. Because the executives always knew that to keep *SportsCenter* fresh we had to continually push the envelope.

Those ESPN suits got—well before I did—that anchors with the freedom to make pop-culture references helped appeal to a diverse audience. They understood that when I reference my black fraternity and Rich Eisen references *Seinfeld*, we say to two very different groups: We're speaking to you. They got that that makes for smart business.

Striking that balance wasn't always easy, at first. In my early years at the network, with a bit of a chip on my shoulder, I kept feeling like I had to point out the blind spots of my colleagues when it came to race. Now, I probably did it in ways that I wouldn't today. I tended to be a little more in-your-face back then—the curse of youth.

I'm always aware of being a black man. You can't help but be. At one point, we were doing a story on former Cowboys receiver Michael Irvin when he had been arrested. It wasn't even my story, but I read the script, which pointed out that he'd worn a mink coat to court. I was hot. "Why say he was wearing a mink coat?" I asked the producer.

"Because he was wearing a mink coat" came the reply.

"But that has nothing to do with anything," I said, probably raising my voice a little. We can be accurate *and* wrong. Because highlighting that detail played into Super Fly stereotypes that aren't fair. We went around about it. Whenever someone claims to be color-blind—black or white—I'm suspicious. Because it's impossible to be unaffected by race—it's all around us every day. I was kind of edgy about pointing that out. But it was important to me to raise the issue so that people started really thinking about the choices they made.

Once, a couple of my boys and I were standing in a hallway,

talking. A white colleague walked by and said, "Hey, it looks like a party."

It stopped me. "Hey, man," I said. "Why isn't it a summit?"

He looked confused.

"Really," I said. "Why's it gotta be a party? How many times do three white guys stand around in the halls of a corporate place? Walk by three brothers, and it's a party?"

Here's the thing. Before you think I was being oversensitive, black men get this kind of thing every day. Little asides that contribute to, rather than break down, stereotypes. And what's so interesting about ESPN is that that kind of thinking has no place in the vision of Skipper and Walsh. The executives have always stood for the most diverse workplace imaginable—which also happened to be in their business self-interest.

One coordinating producer didn't get it. Someone once showed me the post-show reports he gave to the executives, and he killed me a lot of the time. I remember what he'd say whenever I hosted with another black anchor: "They were having too much fun." He never said that about Berman or Kilborn, whose goal had always been to host a comedy show. (Craig went on to precede Jon Stewart as the host of *The Daily Show* before getting his own late-night network talk show.)

Again, this producer wasn't a high-level guy and he wasn't there long. I'm sure he showed his colors in a lot of ways. It was clear to me that his view of the world was out of step with ESPN's, because I knew what the executives stood for.

I rarely watched *Seinfeld*. But Rich Eisen did. When we co-hosted *SportsCenter*, he'd make references to lines from the show that many viewers knew and understood. I'd make references to what I watched instead: *New York Undercover*, the show on Fox that starred Malik Yoba and Michael DeLorenzo as undercover cops—the first police procedural to star two men of color.

Whenever I'd show highlights of Bobby Phills—who played for the Charlotte Hornets and would later tragically die in a car accident—I'd pay him his props as a fellow Alpha man by shouting what we shout: "1-9-0-6!" It was a reference to the date of our fraternity's founding.

"What did that mean?" a producer asked once.

I got that he had to ask—they have to protect the brand. Even though I felt like joking, "Dude, I'm not secretly saying something about hookers and drugs," I played it straight. "It's a fraternity reference," I said.

"Well," he said, "if you're going to make a fraternity reference, why not do something like *Animal House*?"

"Because I didn't *live Animal House*," I said. I got where he was coming from: Not even half the audience was going to get the reference. But I made the argument that there *is* an audience that *will* get it. Alpha is the first and largest black fraternity, and it's worth something to have its alums watching *SportsCenter* and thinking to themselves, probably for the first time, "Wow, *SportsCenter* is talking to *me*."

In the early 2000s, I came to see how important the diversity of these references was to the success of *SportsCenter*. You had the cultural observations of Boomer, Olbermann, Patrick, Kilborn, Eisen, and me. Add into that mix the Canadian flare of John Saunders, the astuteness of Mike Tirico, the class of Robin Roberts, the high-mindedness of Bob Ley, the hockey wisdom of Steve Levy, the free flow of Scott Van Pelt, and the silliness of

Linda Cohn—man, you're touching everybody out there. Potentially every viewer will feel at one point or another that ESPN is reflecting his or her world. ESPN is one of the best examples of why diversity works—because it has always made *SportsCenter* a better show and ESPN a better network.

But none of that would have mattered if tuning in to *SportsCenter* wasn't seen as cool. For all their brilliance, the smartest thing the suits at ESPN did was hire the Portland, Oregon, ad agency Wieden+Kennedy to write and produce commercials that sold the show as *the* meeting place of the sports world. Wieden+Kennedy were the guys behind Nike's iconic "Just Do It" ad campaign—and they'd make *SportsCenter* just as iconic. I knew their commercials had broken new ground when I'd be at a game and pro athletes—I'm talking big-name stars—would come up to me and be, like, "Yo, man, how do I get into one of your commercials?"

"I don't know, man, that's not my department," I'd say. "Have your agent make some phone calls."

The Wieden+Kennedy team was brilliant. They wrote these subtle scripts and filmed them in the most deadpan ways. I'd always acted, but my experience had been in theater—where you have to play it big and loud. Here, I learned, less was more. Playing smaller made the scene more subtle.

My first one featured me and Kenny Mayne tutoring then rookies Kobe Bryant and Keyshawn Johnson on how to handle the media. Kobe and Keyshawn played all meek, totally against type, and Kenny and I were in their faces like drill sergeants, cursing and yelling at them to shout out, "I'm the man!" When the ad ran, of course, I knew the curse words would be bleeped, so I cussed up a storm—something I wouldn't do today. There was no Internet to speak of back then.

Another early one was of me whistling and washing my hands in the men's room. You hear a flush and a coworker comes out of the stall and exits. Then you hear a flush and a jockey comes out of another stall and exits. Then you hear another flush and a *horse* comes out of a stall and exits; my expression is briefly puzzled, before I return to whistling and washing, while the words "This is SportsCenter" appear on the screen. That one took a while to shoot because the horse decided to do some of his business right on the bathroom floor.

Three of my favorites featured me with my man Scott Van Pelt. One had Big Ben Roethlisberger saving people from our building while a fire alarm blared. I'm outside watching this with Van Pelt, and I say, "Does he know this is a drill?"

One that didn't air a whole lot had me and Van Pelt dressed in our designer suits backstage, just off the *SportsCenter* set. We're jittery, like we're athletes waiting to come charging out for the player intros. We're warming up: "One-two, one-two. Get ready. One-two, one-two." We're dapping each other, getting pumped. Then it's time. We rip off our suits like they're warm-ups— underneath, we have the same exact suit. We run onto the set.

The one that was just genius in its subtlety took place in the cafeteria—Van Pelt and I are behind Arnold Palmer as he first puts lemonade into his glass and then follows it with iced tea. It was Arnold Palmer making an . . . Arnold Palmer. We just looked at each other, like: You seeing what I see?

Another one finds me saying that every so often there are rain delays. Then you see a leak from a pipe above our set—and a grounds crew coming out and laying down tarp. "You just hope it lets up," I deadpan.

Rich Eisen and I actually wrote one—I'm not sure if it ever aired. We were shooting a bunch of ads and the director said, "We'd like to shoot one more, a Christmas thing. Any ideas?"

So Rich and I came up with something. We're in the newsroom, with some sappy holiday music playing in the background, and I hand him a gift: "Hey, man, I got you something." He opens the present and it's an earpiece, like we wear on-air. "Go ahead, try it on," I say. He puts it in his ear. "It's a perfect fit," he says. "How'd you know?"

Then he stands up and we exchange the most awkward-looking guy hug imaginable. Just like at our day jobs, we were free to be part of the creative process behind the ads.

What is so great about the "This is SportsCenter" campaign is that it makes being at Bristol the fantasy. In the ads, everyone from Roger Federer to Tiger Woods is hanging out at ESPN. To me and my coanchors, we were broadcasting scores and highlights from a sleepy Connecticut town. To Wieden+Kennedy, what we did had a lot of romance to it. They sold us as the stand-in for the American male sports fantasy. Pretty cool.

WHEN SYDNI WAS BORN, in October 1999, I continued a ritual that started when Taelor was born, and that continues in some form to this day. Every night, I'd sneak into their rooms and watch them sleep.

This is my purpose, I'd think, looking at them. *This is the only purpose I have. Protecting these two sleeping girls.*

It probably sounds like some stupid tough-guy thing, but every night I'd have the same thought: *You can't come in here and hurt them.* I didn't even know who the "you" was—but I knew that this is why I was here. And I'd carry on these conversations with whoever was out there trying to do my babies harm. *You'll have to go through me and kill me. Not on my watch. This is my watch.*

Sometimes I'd sit in the rocking chair in their room and listen to the hum of their breathing while consciously sending out these warnings. *They're sleeping in my house, now. You don't get to hurt them. Not here, not tonight. This is why I'm here. If you want to hurt them, I will end your life. Or die trying.*

Even now, I open Sydni's door at night and watch her sleep. Taelor, too, when she's home from college. I'll watch for a while, thanking God, and then I'll kiss each on her forehead. Because even though Taelor may not call as often as I want her to and Sydni will roll her eyes when I think I'm being one cool dad, I stare at them at night and . . . they're still my little angels.

They're very close, my girls, and fiercely loyal to each other. Taelor is the protective big sister. Even when she was younger—she's five years Sydni's senior—she'd come down on me if I was too tough for her liking on her baby sister.

"You do not get to speak to her like that," Taelor would reprimand me.

"I'm talking to your sister," I'd say. "Stay out of it."

She would not back down. "No, you do *not* get to talk to her like that," she'd insist.

What an interesting dynamic as a parent. Part of me wants to say, *I'm your father—you don't get to talk to me like that.* But another part of me is, like, *Damn right, girl. You battle anybody who you feel is messing with your sister. You battle and you don't give up the fight.*

When Taelor would stand up to me I'd secretly swell with pride. I may have to pretend to be stern with her, but inside I'm thinking: *I love your moxie right now. Your parent is sitting here blasting you and you're, like, "Pffft, bring it, 'cause I'm gonna bring it right back at you."* When she'd fight me, even as a strong-willed six-year-old, I kinda loved it—because it showed me how tough she was.

Kim and I separated in 2005, and the divorce was final in 2007. Marriage is hard, man. Even when you think you're doing your best to keep it together, it doesn't always work out. Sydni was five, Taelor was ten, and it ripped their life apart. Funny, I'd always been so dead set on protecting them, but I couldn't protect them from this. What they knew their whole life as safe and secure was no more. When you divorce, you change your children's lives forever. I don't know about other parents, but I'll never get over that. My ex-wife and I forever altered our girls' sense of security.

They were both more confident before the divorce, especially Taelor. When they were little, I always thought Taelor would be the more outgoing one. But it turns out she's not as social as Sydni. They're both highly sensitive. Sydni hides her sensitivity behind a blank stare more than Taelor.

After the separation, I moved into my condo and I hurriedly furnished it so it would feel like home to the girls. My ex and I shared joint custody; I'd get the girls three nights a week. On Tuesdays, I'd pick Sydni up after school and we'd go to West Hartford Center, the closest cool downtown to us. Sydni took tae kwon do and Taelor took dance lessons there. Sydni and I would hang out at Starbucks. I'd get a coffee and she'd have her "yellow milk"—vanilla milk, but she was used to it in the yellow container from the grocery store. She was a lot like me as a kid—she had energy to burn. She'd bounce around Starbucks like that Tasmanian Devil in the cartoons. We'd take coffee stirrers and use them as drumsticks and have our own little jam session at the table.

Those are some of my best memories, Sydni and I hanging out every week at Starbucks. Today, she's fifteen and doesn't seem as jazzed by the memory as I am. "Hey, Syd," I'll say, "want to go to Starbucks for a jam session?"

"No, Dad," she'll say, sighing.

It's funny, watching them grow. Parents tend to label their kids—the smart one, the jock—but I found it interesting just how both of my girls defied expectations. Taelor started dancing at four years old and became a very eclectic kid. She never dressed like the other girls; she dresses more like a struggling New York artist. She never had a ton of friends but always had an adult's sense of humor. She is a great writer and dancer. Once, her dance company won platinum—the highest score—in an intense competition. I can still remember her jumping up and down—pure joy. Is there any feeling on earth better than what you feel when you watch your kid triumph at something?

Taelor didn't play sports, but I know she was a naturally gifted athlete. In eighth grade she played on the volleyball team. She had never played the game. I went to her first game and she didn't know what she was doing. As a parent, when you watch your kid flailing around like that, you're, like, *Eeesh*. I couldn't get to another game for a couple of weeks. Meantime, Taelor said: "The coach has to play everyone, and I'm one of the best players." I didn't say anything, but I thought: *My God. She's delusional. Dude, you're not one of the best players.*

Well, I went to the next game and I didn't know who she was. She was all over the court, running down every ball, setting up her taller teammates for spikes, barking commands. My jaw was at my knees. In two weeks she had totally picked up the game and *was* one of the best players on the team. Still, that didn't compel her to stick with it or to take up other sports. She was too interested in art and film and dance.

Sydni is more social than Taelor. She's constantly texting her friends. She has gifts playing soccer that other girls don't have. She's fast as all get-out. She turns on the jets and she's gone. And she is a ridiculous singer.

When Sydni was little we found out she was allergic to peanuts and tree nuts. Dealing with that has always been a part of her life, and I've always been proud of how she does it. She'd go away with the soccer team and have to bring her own snacks. She'd have to check with school cafeteria workers about the ingredients of menu items and with other girls' moms about snacks brought in from home for special occasions. It was a pain, but she always accepted it as just part of her life. She never felt sorry for herself. We'd go to a restaurant, and, as young as six years old, she'd ask to speak to the chef: "I'm allergic to peanuts and tree nuts," she'd say. "Can you make sure whatever I have has no peanuts or tree nuts? And can you make my food on a dedicated free spot?"

Most nights, I'd get back home at two or three in the morning after *SportsCenter.* Sydni, at about four years old, would get up in the middle of every night and walk all the way down the hall to my bedroom to get me so I could walk her back down the hall to the bathroom so she could pee. She'd climb up on the toilet, and I'd just stroke her hair or scratch her back before walking her back into her room, where I'd rock her back to sleep in the rocking chair. I remember looking at us, me and my little girl, in the mirror, rocking slowly, and I remember being so, so tired . . . but I also remember saying to myself: *Don't ever say no. Don't ever be too tired for this.*

Because I knew that someday it was going to stop. Some night, I was going to get home from a draining night on the *SportsCenter* set and I wouldn't hear the pitter-patter of those little feet coming down the hall. I don't remember the night it happened, but when it ended—it ended.

At my condo, Taelor and Sydni had a bunk bed in their room, but Sydni would sleep with me in my room. People who don't have kids tend to react like "Oh, that's weird." But if you have kids, you get it. Around when she was eight, I started wondering, *When is she going to stop? When is she supposed to stop?*

A friend of mine told me: "You'll know. *She'll* know." And then one day, when she was nine, she said, "Dad, I don't think I want to sleep in the bed with you anymore."

And I said, "Okay." It was the most natural thing. But, man, did I miss having her there. People always say, when you have a baby, just wait until your kid walks or talks or plays sports. No. Don't look ahead to anything. Enjoy every moment in the present, man, because these moments end. And once they end they don't come back again. One day, my little girl stopped coming down the hall for me to walk her to the bathroom and then rock her back to sleep. One day my baby girl decided it didn't feel right to sleep in her dad's bed anymore. I got lucky: She told me so. Usually you don't know when these moments end. You just know *I don't get to do that anymore.*

I don't know how, but I knew this. That these moments end, so you'd better soak up every one of them. You soak it up because you don't get to take them to pee in the middle of the night forever. You don't get them kicking the covers off you at three in the morning forever.

I DIDN'T KNOW HERM EDWARDS, but I knew that booming coach's voice of his. It was January 2002, he was the head coach of the New York Jets, and I cold-called him with an idea: I wanted to come to minicamp as a player, with ESPN cameras documenting how I did.

"Can you *play*?" he asked. I could tell he was amused.

"Yes, coach, I played high school ball and club ball at UNC, which was like D II level football," I said.

"What position you play?"

"Wide receiver, coach."

There was a pause. "Aw, what the hell, c'mon up," he said. "This oughta be fun."

What I didn't tell Coach Edwards was that I'd been playing in a league in Waterbury, Connecticut, for about five years. It was contact flag football, live-speed, full blocking from the waist up. We'd play nine-on-nine with two refs. Each team had multiple former college players. One guy had been a wideout at Division II Southern Connecticut State, a 6'4" receiver who ran a legit 4.4 forty. For three straight years he lasted deep into NFL training camps. Two years in a row, we watched him catch a preseason touchdown pass only to then get cut. The next week, I'd be lining up against him—and holding my own.

It's interesting why he didn't end up making the league. At Southern Connecticut, no one played press coverage against him due to his speed. So he didn't know how to handle NFL bump-and-run coverage. Being the big fish in a little pond in college worked against him because he wasn't used to cornerbacks getting all up in his grill on the line of scrimmage.

Anyway, I'd always wondered just how good I could be at football. Yes, I was doing this for a story. But I was also doing it to test myself and for the pure love of the game. Coach Edwards invited me to the team's OTAs—organized team activities. We'd practice, have team meetings. After going through OTAs, the next step would be participating in minicamp—with my camera crew catching the highs and lows.

In preparation for OTAs, I hit the gym. One of my best buddies in Connecticut is Brian Gallagher, a personal trainer at Farmington Farm Gym. I grabbed a buddy of mine who had set track records at Dartmouth, and we hit Brian's gym every day. I'd run hundreds of pass patterns a day, my buddy trying to check me.

I went to a celebrity golf tournament in Hawaii, where I ran into Drew Brees and LaDainian Tomlinson. They were both with their then girlfriends—now wives. I asked them if they'd work out with me. Talk about a busman's holiday—here are two of the best in the world at what they do, on vacation in Hawaii, and they kindly agree to work me out. Love those dudes to this day.

We found a field, and for two hours it was Drew rifling spirals and LaDainian beating on me, and me beating on LaDainian. I was holding my own running patterns against LaDainian and checking him, which gave me a bit of a swagger that he must have noticed.

"Man, you got cleats on!" LaDainian said. Yeah, I'd come prepared.

"You're a Pro Bowl running back, don't give me any of this 'You got cleats on!'" I said.

That same trip, I got together with Jaguars wide receiver Keenan McCardell. We ran patterns together and spent hours talking receiving.

I felt ready for my first day of OTAs, which took place at Hofstra University. We'd start with conditioning drills and weight lifting, go into a classroom session, and then hit the field for practice. Going in, I expected one of three reactions from the players. Some would be excited to see me. Some would be ticked off that I was there—an interloper. And some would just be skeptical.

Quarterback Chad Pennington was in that first group. My locker was next to his, and when he walked in and saw me his eyes lit up. "Well, okay, man," he said, giving me a bro hug. "I saw the name—was wondering if that was you. That's cool."

I could tell wideout Laveranues Coles was a skeptic. One of the linebackers—I didn't even know who it was, just that he was a big boy—walked by us and said to Laveranues: "This ain't no place for reporters. I bet he won't come across the middle."

I said, loud enough for others to hear, "I'm right here." I just wanted everyone to know: If you want to say stuff, say it to my face.

Once we got in the gym I could tell Laveranues was starting to come around. He saw that I was willing to work. In the classroom session, we worked on a curl pattern, how to drive the cornerback off, plant, and come back. And then we went out onto the field.

There, I was timed running my fastest-ever 40-yard dash, 4.55. I'd been timed at 4.6 in college. Not bad for a thirty-six-year-old. There were some murmurings of "atta boy" and "way to go" after that; I was winning over at least some of the skeptics.

Next, we were going to catch passes off the JUGS machine. I'd never caught off a JUGS machine. I was running a wideout pattern. I'd always learned that you put your hands up to catch the ball at the last possible moment—you don't want to be waiting for the ball with your arms outstretched. The first ball that came to me got on me much faster than I ever would have thought; it was there, past my hands, before I could react. The thud was deafening. The ball hit me square in my left eye, ripping it open. All was quiet.

The ball literally split my eyeball open. The lens and the iris had come out. I remember getting in the shower and thinking, *Man, my eye is messed up*, before being taken to the hospital. I had emergency surgery that night. I was hurt, but also embarrassed. Later, I would read that the wide receivers coach had me ranked sixth of the eight receivers in camp. That, plus my time in the 40, gave me some solace. But that was later. That night, I was

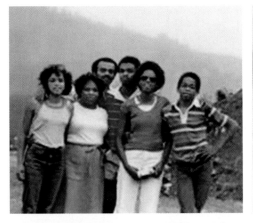

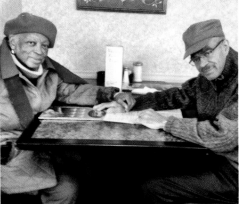

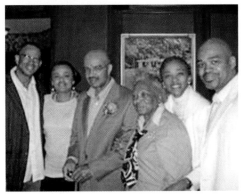

CLOCKWISE FROM TOP LEFT:
The Scotts, late '70s: Synthia, Jackie, Ray, Stephen, Susan, and me. Jackie and Ray Scott modeled a lifelong, loving relationship for all of us. The sibling Scotts wearing our special T-shirts at dinner, ESPYs week 2014: left to right, Stephen, Susan, Synthia, and yours truly. Celebrating our parents' 50th wedding anniversary (2008).

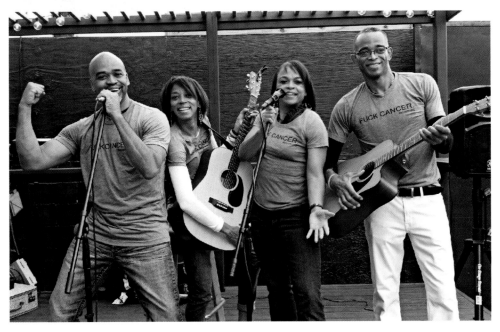

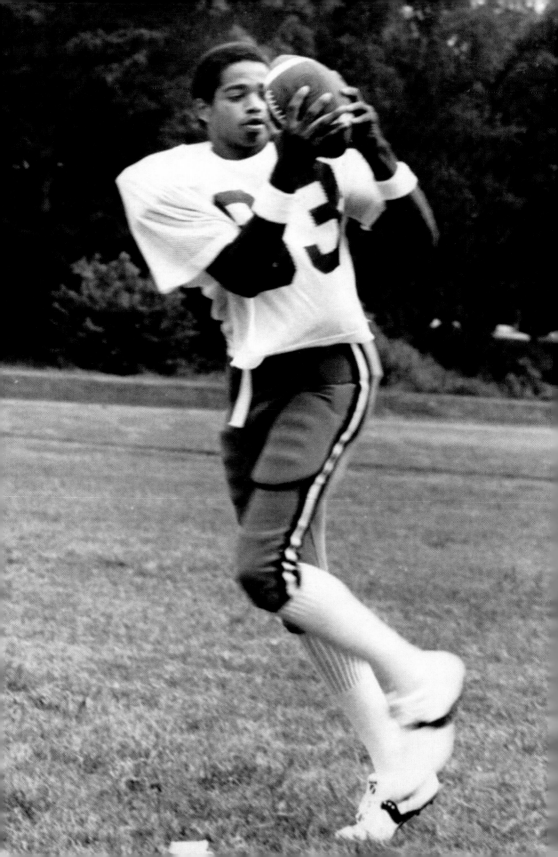

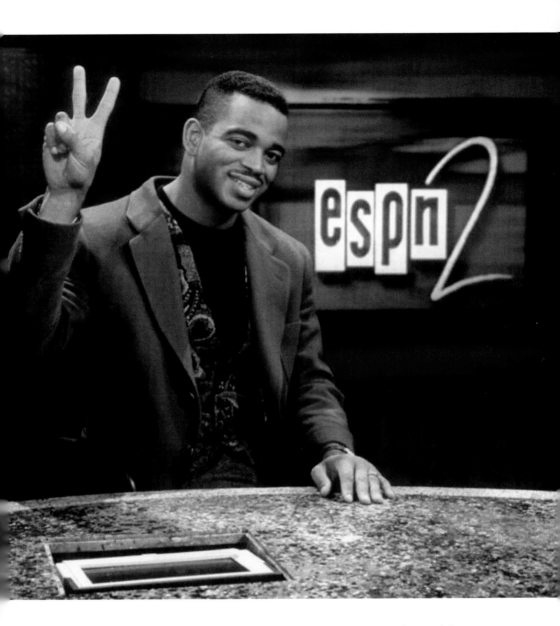

ABOVE: In 1993, I made my debut
on ESPN 2, "The Deuce."

LEFT: My first love: Catching a tight
spiral in stride.

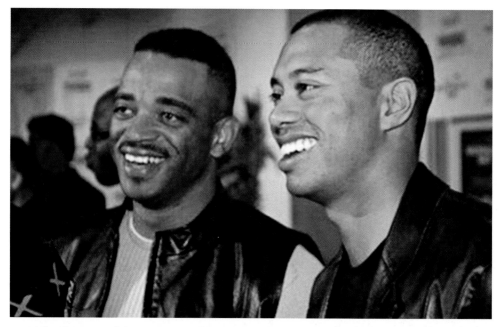

They're two of the greatest athletes in history, but when I get together with Tiger Woods and Michael Jordan, our realest moments come when we talk about our kids.

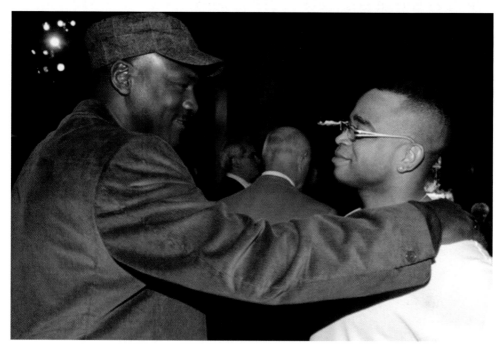

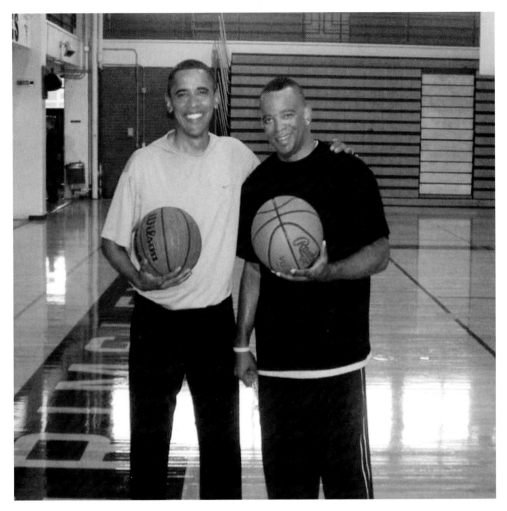

In 2008, candidate Obama took me to the hardcourt house of pain.
Dude's got game.

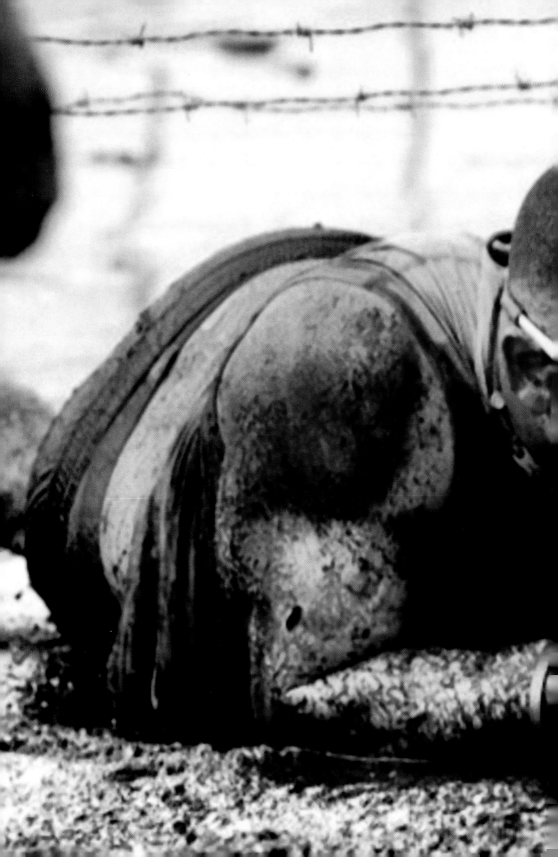

Three days after a chemo session, I ran a Savage Race five-mile obstacle course through mud, over blockades, and under barbed wire, before swimming in ice cold water.

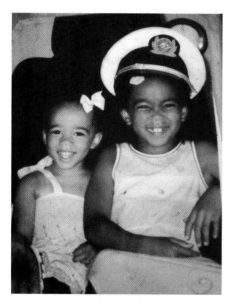

My life changed when these two
knuckleheads came into it. That's
Sydni, left, and Taelor, right. Being a
Dad? Best thing I've ever done.

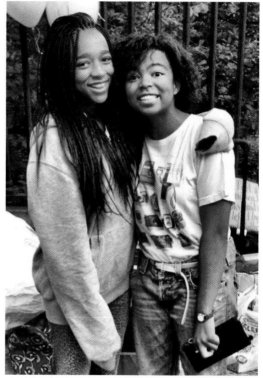

Sydni, left, and Taelor, right. Grown, but still
my baby girls.

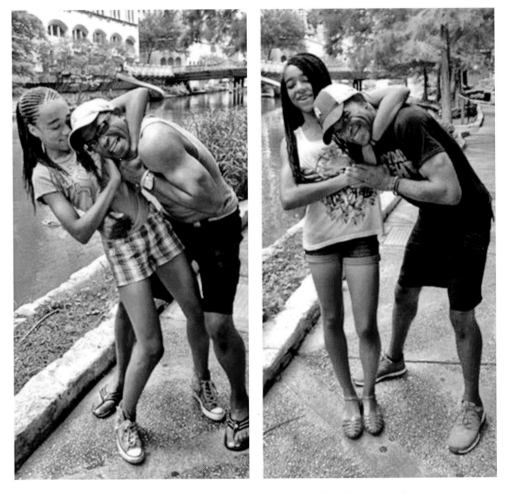

The same pose, a few years apart: Sydni head-locking her ol' man.

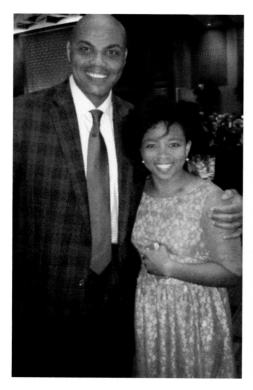

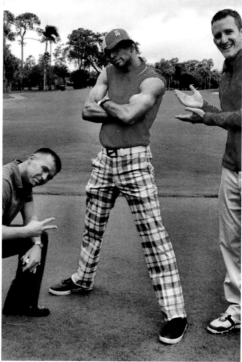

CLOCKWISE FROM TOP LEFT:

Charles Barkley and Taelor share a birthday: Not a year goes by that Charles doesn't call her, just like he regularly checks in with me to make sure I'm holding up. Clowning on the links with my boys: That's Brian Gallagher on the left and Doug Ulman on the right. Kristin and I would say that life consists of two dates with a dash in between— and our job was to make the most of the dash. Man, did we.

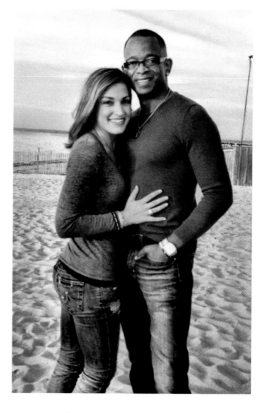

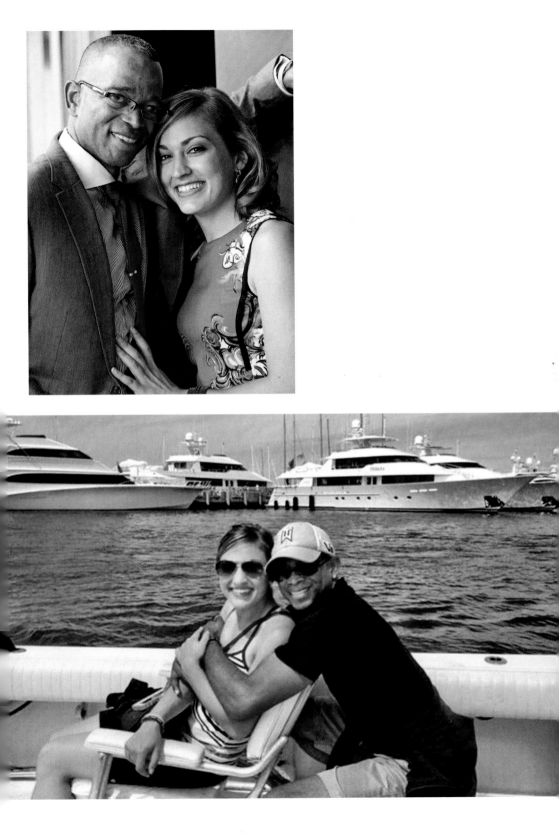

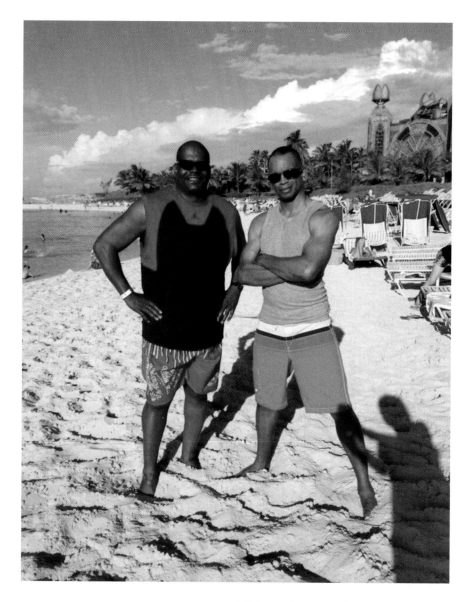

ABOVE: With my longtime best friend, Fred Tindal, during one of our annual Daddy/Daughter Week getaways.

RIGHT: Bring it, chemo!

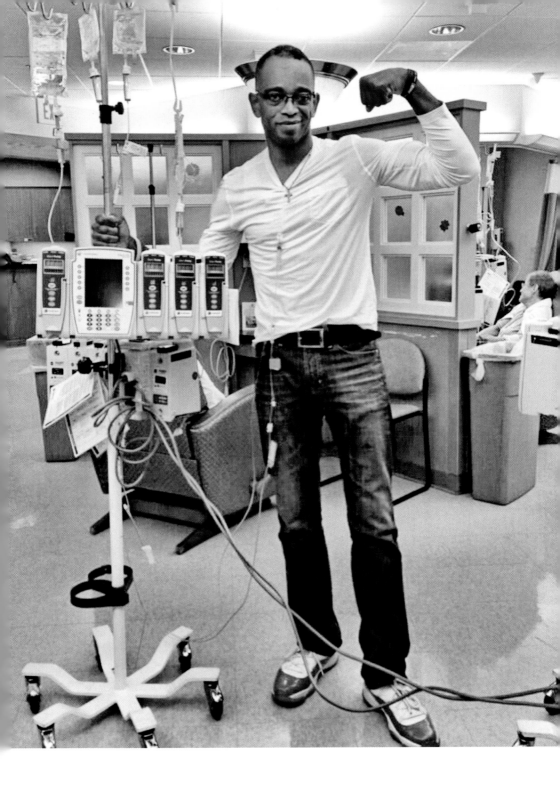

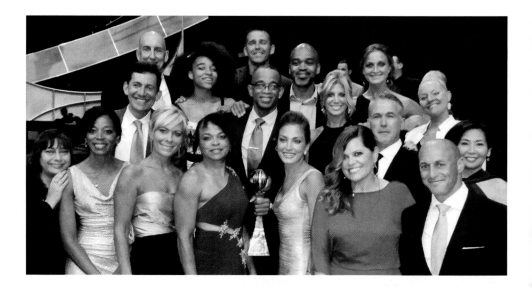

ABOVE: My peeps, sharing the 2014 ESPYs with me. Left to right: Bottom row, Jackie Harris, Susan, Deedee Mills, Synthia, Kristin, Amy Bartlett, Matthew Vujovich. Middle: Gerry Matalon, Sydni, Me, Laura Okmin, Mike Hagerty, Barb Lee, Shannon McGauley. Top: Scott Organ, Brian Gallagher, Stephen, Jackie Barry.

RIGHT: Robin Roberts gets it, because she's been there. She's not only been a friend, but a shoulder to lean on.

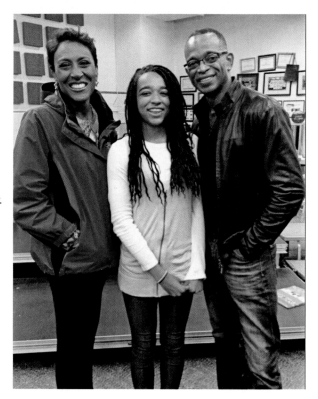

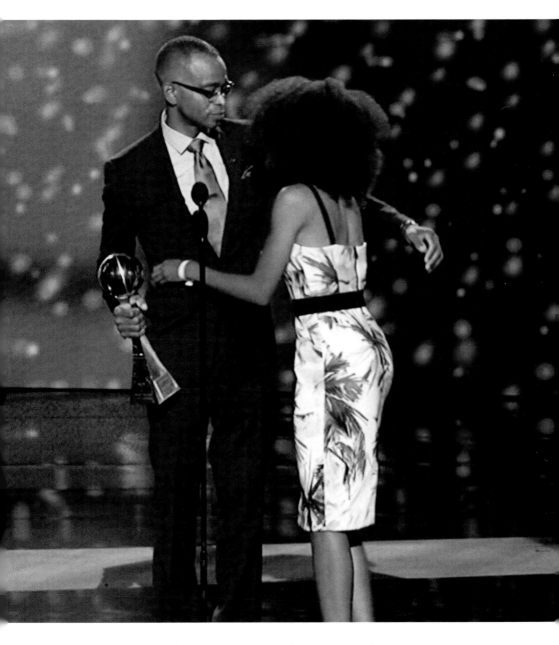

My littlest angel, Sydni, on the ESPYs stage with me as I get the Jimmy V Perseverance Award. "This is why I needed you here," I told her, as we hugged tightly.

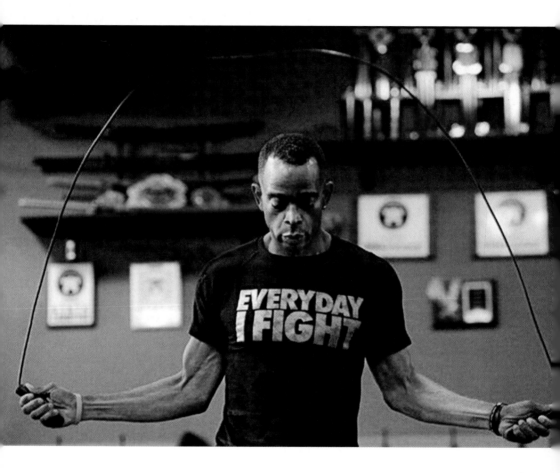

down. Besides worrying whether I'd have my eyesight come the next day, I was bummed because this was not how the day was supposed to play out. What's that saying? Man plans, and God laughs.

You know about my history of eye trouble. It's gonna read like a litany of bad luck, and you're going to wonder why this dude keeps playing sports, since many of my injuries have happened on a field or court. What can I say? It's what I do.

I'd had a cornea transplant in my right eye in 1983 that didn't take; they did it again, but my vision in that eye never got back to where it had been. Two years later, I had a successful cornea transplant in my left eye. From then on, my left eye was my good eye—I wore a contact lens that gave me 20/25 vision in it.

In 1989, playing pickup basketball in Raleigh, I was on the sideline waiting for next when someone whipped a pass that hit me in my right eye. It hurt like hell, but I shrugged it off and played. Two days later, I started seeing stars. The next day, what looked like a curtain came up from the bottom of my vision. In other words, the bottom half of my vision just went dark. A detached retina. My eye doctor stapled the retina back together and put a water bubble in my eye to keep it together. Two years later, in Orlando, I saw the curtain again and knew what it was: The retina had detached all by itself. This time I went to Duke—yeah, Tar Heels suck it up and go to Duke when it's medically necessary—for a laser reattachment.

But now with my left eye—my good eye—shattered, I was worried for my career. My right eye had 20/35 vision, but now the vision in my left eye was horrible. On top of that, over the next year, I battled glaucoma. My eye pressure kept getting higher and higher, and I must have had six or eight surgeries to decrease it.

Almost a year to the day after the Jets debacle, I went to Vegas for Tiger's annual golf tournament. I wasn't wearing glasses, and I had a contact lens in my right eye. I was meeting one of my boys in a casino lobby. We saw each other and did that brother high-five hug. Only, as he came to me, his pinky inadvertently went right into my left eye. I heard it pop. It was one a.m. in Vegas and I knew what had happened. Another rupture. Tiger was kind enough to let my brother Stephen and me use his jet, a Cessna Citation X—the fastest civilian jet in the sky—to fly to Johns Hopkins in Baltimore. I had another cornea transplant. A year later, another one.

All this time, the real danger was the glaucoma. The pressure kept building and building, and finally, my optic nerve gave out. By 2004, I was effectively blind in my left eye—which had been, up until a couple of years before that, my good eye. Again: Man plans, God laughs.

I remember my eye doctor telling me I shouldn't be playing football. And the truth is, I would have played a lot more football in my life were it not for my eye troubles. But, sorry, I'm not *not* going to play football. Now when I play I wear protective goggles. They offer some protection, but if you get punched in the eye you're not going to be completely protected. So I try to be smart about it.

"Anyone who's had the same things that have happened to me, what are they going to do?" I told Kristin. "Sit on the couch forever?"

"Some people do," she said.

"I don't think most would," I said. "I think most people would just live their life."

"Most people wouldn't play football again," she said, smiling.

"That's probably true," I said. "But I'm not going to compromise on my quality of life. Maybe that's stupid."

But Kristin, God bless her, wasn't hearing that. "Some would call it stupid, but you would probably call them stupid if they never did anything for the rest of their lives because they had eye problems or cancer or whatever," she said.

If my left eye gets hit even a little bit again, it can rupture very easily because there's nothing left in there but cornea. The things that give it strength—the iris, the lens—are long gone. We were in Myrtle Beach, South Carolina, just walking along, and someone right in front of me shot out his arm. Because I don't see out of my left eye, it doesn't close. The guy hit my glasses, my eye was wide open, and the glasses went right into my eye. My eye-print was left on the glasses. I was afraid it was another rupture, but it wasn't.

When I'm in bed, I sleep on the right, so that if I'm looking at Kristin my left eye is on the pillow. Why? So my right eye can pick up anything coming at me. Why tell you this? Because if I'm in danger of another rupture while walking on the beach or while lying in my bed, I know enough now to know that I'm not in control of what's going to happen. Remember: Man plans, God laughs. So what the hell? Might as well do what I love. Might as well play some football.

CHAPTER SEVEN

I WON'T BE HERE FOR MY DAUGHTERS

t was supposed to be a laugher. But sports—a lot like life, as I was about to find out—don't always play out as expected. On Sunday, November 25, 2007, I was on my way to Pittsburgh for a *Monday Night Football* matchup the next night between the 7-3 Steelers, a Super Bowl contender led by Big Ben Roethlisberger, and the lowly 0-10 Miami Dolphins.

When *Monday Night Football* moved to ESPN in 2006, I was asked to cohost the ninety-minute pregame show with Chris Berman. Boomer from the studio, me in the field. Of course, no one had to ask. Monday night games have always held a special place for me. I grew up on it, getting home from football practice, scarfing down a quick meal, rushing through my homework before kickoff. Games would go so late, it wasn't until high school that my parents let me stay up to watch the second half. I soaked it all in: Howard Cosell's opinions, Dandy Don Meredith's singing (*"Turn out the lights, the party's over"*), and Frank Gifford's play-by-play. Talk about iconic television; those guys broke new ground and influenced the entire country. It was appointment television. That's why, when *GQ* called me the "hip-hop Howard Cosell," I was honored.

Now here I was, same broadcast. While many saw me, as the *GQ* mention might have implied, as little more than a young upstart, I actually obsessively prepared for these games. On the plane that Sunday, I went over my stack of notes from around the league. I read every stat and checked out what each coach was saying about that week's game. In live television, you don't want any surprises.

The Steelers were coming off a disappointing overtime loss the previous week to the New York Jets, 19–16. So they'd be looking to make up for letting one slip away. Pittsburgh would be playing at home, where they were 5-0, and on Monday night—where they were undefeated in twelve appearances. I was feeling a rout coming on.

But something else was coming on, too. My stomach hurt all day. I kept feeling like I had to go to the bathroom—and I'm not talking about number one. I was in pain all night at the hotel. I wondered if it was something I ate. Some bug?

The next day, I drank tea to try to settle my stomach. I rested in my room. I even skipped my regular Monday morning workout. Nothing worked. In fact, the pain might have been getting worse. Finally, around lunchtime, I went to the hospital.

After some tests, a doctor told me I had appendicitis. "It's best that we take it out, now," he said.

"Can I at least go back to Connecticut and have it done there?"

He thought for a moment. "Well, it hasn't ruptured yet," he said. "How quickly can you get back there?"

"I'll charter a flight right away, and I promise I'll go straight to the hospital," I said.

Once I had his blessing, I called ESPN and my hospital back

in Connecticut. It was all set up. But what's that I was saying about God laughing? There was a hellacious rain and lightning storm leveling the Northeast. All commercial flights were grounded. In fact, the game was being delayed. I chartered a flight and went to the FBO—a fixed-base operator, which is like a service station for private aircrafts. They told us we could take off, but that we might have to be rerouted to Wilkes-Barre, Pennsylvania.

I got nothing against Wilkes-Barre, but if I was about to be cut open, Pittsburgh seemed to be the better choice. So back to the hospital I went. Late that night, I had my appendix taken out.

The next day, Kim, my ex-wife, flew in. We were still close, going so far as to take family vacations together with the kids. That morning, one of the doctors told me I should be able to go home by the next morning—Wednesday.

On Wednesday morning, though, no one came to tell me anything. Lunchtime came and went. I felt okay. I joked with a nurse: Had they forgotten about me? Bureaucracy, right?

On Wednesday evening, the doctor who had performed the surgery came into my room. "Things just got more complicated," he said.

There was a pause. "We biopsied your appendix, and it's cancerous."

The word landed with a thud.

I must have looked confused. "You have cancer," the doctor said.

I wish I could explain this moment: It's a sledgehammer to your gut, to your chest. It's a feeling of pressure, like you're about to burst all over. Funny, before that moment, whenever I'd hear of someone getting diagnosed with cancer, I'd think: *Oh, that's tough, but maybe there's medicine, maybe there's a good chance of survival.*

When it's you, there's zero of that. There were two thoughts that occurred to me, one right on top of the other—a lightning-fast, devastating combination:

I'm going to die.

And then, worse:

I won't be here for my daughters.

I don't have words for how deep and profound those two thoughts are together. But they have a physical impact. I loved the impact of hitting and being hit on the football field. This, though, hurt in a far different way: I felt it over my whole body and I couldn't will it away.

I won't be here for my daughters.

It was this last thought that started bouncing around my head—I couldn't stop it. Meantime, the doc was talking. "You're going to need more surgery," he said. "And we're not talking about in a few days. Really, really soon. We need to go in and take out whatever is close to your appendix. If your appendix is cancerous, there's a good chance it's somewhere else in that vicinity."

He was talking about going back in first thing the next morning.

I won't be here for my daughters.

"No, no, no," I said. "I have to see my daughters."

"Time is really of the essence here—" the doc said.

I won't be here for my daughters.

"I have to see my daughters," I said. My memory of this exchange is shaky; I may have been repeating this over and over, like a mantra. Finally, the colorectal surgeon came to confer with us, and he mentioned that he knew Dr. Jeffrey Milsom at New York–Presbyterian Hospital, whom he described as *the* man when it came to cases like this. A colorectal Michael Jordan, in other words. He said he'd call him.

I wish I could say I was processing this information. I just kept thinking about my girls—that I was abandoning them. Even when I was conversing with the doctors, I wasn't really present. I wasn't feeling fear—not yet, at least. I was numb. Most people who are diagnosed with cancer are aware of its possibility before learning they have it. They've undergone a test—a CT scan, a mammogram, something—that they know might bring them the news.

Not me. I was having my appendix out—only to learn of my diagnosis upon waking up. What did I know of cancer? Not much. You get it and you die. That's what I knew—or thought I knew. Living in CancerWorld is always a touch surreal, but those first days were especially so. Time has stopped, while the world keeps swirling around you.

Within an hour, I was on the phone with Dr. Milsom. He's a leading innovator in using high-tech, minimally invasive technologies to perform colon and rectal surgeries. The dude has published four books and more than 250 papers, presentations, and educational videos, and has been invited to perform surgery in more than fifteen countries.

But he wasn't one of those coolly detached docs. You could tell the guy really cared. He was in his mid-fifties and spoke softly. "I honestly try to say to myself every morning," he says in a video that's posted online, "'What would it be like if that were me that's going to be that recipient of care? . . .' When I'm operating on a patient, I'm thinking about their kids that are out in the waiting room. I'm saying, 'By God, I'm going to find a way to fix this, to make this person better.'"

"Listen," he said when we first spoke. "I'm going out of the country on Saturday. If you can get here in time, I can do the surgery on Friday and my team will care for you after that, until I get back." There was a sense of calm and confidence in his voice.

We had a plan. I called my bosses. True to who they are, they chartered a plane for me. I was going home. Thursday night, on the eve of my surgery, the girls would come over. I still couldn't stop thinking about them. About what I was *doing* to them, even though—rationally—I knew *I* hadn't *done* anything to them. I'd have to sit them down. And I'd have to tell them. Our lives were about to change.

By the way, in a delayed start due to the weather, the Steelers beat the Dolphins 3–0 in monsoon-like conditions on a late field goal. I couldn't care less.

IN THE DAYS that followed, there were moments of confusion—how had this happened? There's no history of cancer in my family. I didn't live near any toxic waste dumpsites. I felt physically strong. Could I really be sick? It was hard to believe.

Once you're told you have it, cancer is never not with you. My life was now forever divided between the before and the after of my diagnosis. I'd look at people walking by and I'd think: *You don't have cancer.* It wasn't said with envy—like I said before, I never had a *Why me?* moment, in part because I still felt incredibly lucky to have this life: my family, my girls, my job. No, I'd say it to myself as a simple matter of fact when I looked at another dad on the sidelines at soccer practice or when I stood in line behind an errand-running mom at Starbucks: *You don't have cancer.*

Look at these people, I'd think. *Eating and drinking, laughing. He's healthy. Look how relaxed she looks.* As the days turned to weeks, the weeks to months, and the months now to years of this mental and physical Kabuki dance between me and these radical cells in my body, I came to realize what I was really doing making these observations: I was noting the innocence of others. And, on some level, I was mourning my loss of the same.

I would never have that again. That carefree, total immersion in simple moments. From now on, whenever I laughed, it would no longer be an innocent laugh; it would instead be tinged with the bittersweet fear that I had only so many laughs remaining. That now there were finite numbers left to me: a finite number of laughs, of hours spent with the girls, of days.

The fear rose in me, became my constant companion. Though one of the doctors in Pittsburgh cautioned me not to, I Googled "appendiceal cancer" once I got back to the condo in Connecticut.

Awareness of different forms of cancer has grown in recent years. There's been the pink-ribbon campaign for breast cancer and Katie Couric's televised colonoscopy to call attention to colon cancer. But I had never heard of cancer of the appendix.

Only 600 to 1,000 Americans are diagnosed with it each year. In 1993, it received a moment's attention in the news when Audrey Hepburn passed away from it.

There are no symptoms. It's usually discovered during the course of abdominal surgery, as in my case. About 1 percent of all appendectomies result in a cancer diagnosis. Since it usually has no symptoms, by the time it is discovered the cancer has likely spread. It has no known cause. There are no lifestyle changes you can make to avoid it.

God bless the Internet. In my job, I can pull up any stat or video clip. Remember when we were kids, we had to actually go to the library to find information? I don't regret our 24/7 access to information. But as I sat at my kitchen table, surfing the Web, I felt my anxiety level rising. Like the initial hit of those words— "You have cancer"—I physically felt the fear building up. Let's face it, man, there ain't a whole lotta good stories on the Internet. With every click, I ran across another stat or another anecdote that made me feel scared, worried, anxious.

Yet I couldn't stop clicking. I learned that 41 percent of Americans will be diagnosed with cancer during their lifetime; 21 percent will die of the disease. Nevertheless, a report for the President's Cancer Panel concluded that research on the environmental causes of cancer has been underfunded. As for my own type, the five-year survival rates of appendiceal cancer danced across my screen; with each one, I felt my blood pressure jump higher. Stage 1: 88%. Stage 2: 75.2%. Stage 3: 37.2%. Stage 4: 25.6%.

I pushed the laptop away, leaned back in my chair, and closed my eyes. This was wrong. The way I was feeling was . . . wrong.

I'm in the information business. My whole professional life has been dedicated to finding stuff out and telling people about it. But the way I was feeling now had me thinking. Maybe there is such a thing as too much information, after all?

SINCE THEY WERE IN CRIBS, I'd always had adult conversations with my girls. I always leveled with them. Taelor and Sydni might have only been twelve and eight, respectively, but I thought they were ready for the most adult conversation of their young lives. As I contemplated it, I started to realize that it wasn't just *my* innocence that would forever be changed.

The girls sat on my bed. Taelor seemed to sense something was wrong. I couldn't tell if Sydni did or not. I was half lying down, wanting to show them that I was relaxed about this—but I also didn't want to totally recline and look too fatigued.

"I've got cancer," I began by saying—getting the hardest part out of the way. As I was still accepting it myself, the words sounded strange to me. Like I was playing a part. Before they could say anything, I continued.

"Listen, we're going to fight this," I said. "I'm going to be strong about it. We're going to have faith, we're going to say prayers, and I'm going to tackle this strong."

There was a pause. "Daddy, are you going to die?" Sydni asked. I remember how wide her eyes looked.

"I could, baby girl," I said. "But we've got the best doctors and I'm going to get the best medicine, and if I do everything I'm supposed to—eat right, take my medicine, rest—you ain't getting rid of me."

I wanted them to know that, as much as I could, I was going to make sure our lives didn't change. "We're going to live our life like we always do," I said. "We're still going to have fun. We're still going to travel, like we always do." In the following weeks, we'd make our annual Christmastime trip to New York, stay at the Plaza Hotel, see the Alvin Ailey dancers, go ice-skating. Between courses of chemo, we'd hop on a plane to visit Orlando and spend spring break in Arizona.

I told them I had surgery the next morning. We'd know more then about the fight we were in. They didn't say much. They gave me hugs and kisses—which felt like medicine.

We prayed. Prayer is an interesting thing. I'm not a loud God Squad guy; when guys imply in interviews that the Lord made them juke that defender and score that touchdown, it tends to rub me wrong. I pray, but I pray for His will to be done—not mine. I acknowledge in every prayer that what I want may not be what He wants.

I know that some patients, given a cancer diagnosis, might pray to get well. That's only natural. Some even start deal making: "God, if you let me beat this, I swear I'll . . ." I've never once gone there: *Hey, get me to remission, and I'll start helping old ladies cross the street.*

Instead, I do what we did that day I first told Taelor and Sydni I had cancer. We prayed for wisdom. We prayed for patience and a sense of calm. We prayed for the strength to handle this upcoming fight.

That's what it was, after all: a fight. I was starting to wrap my head around that. That's when I decided. With visions of those survival rates still flashing before my eyes, I told Dr. Milsom before the surgery: "When I wake up, I want to know what you found and what you did, but I don't want to know what stage I'm in."

He looked puzzled.

"With all due respect, Doc, I'm not going to be interested in how long you *think* I have," I said. It took me a few days, but like an athlete who doesn't read the sports pages in the days leading up to the Super Bowl, I was getting ready to do battle.

CHAPTER EIGHT

NEVER DIE EASY

L et's play word association. Throw the word "tough" my way and a few names instantly come to mind.

One would be Walter Payton. Yes, his nickname was Sweetness, but I always thought that missed an essential part of the guy. In fact, there was speculation that, when he got the nickname while starring at historically black Jackson State University, it was meant sarcastically—because he was such an aggressive player.

When I think of the literal definition of the word "tough"— "strong enough to withstand adverse conditions or rough or careless handling"—I wonder why we don't just put Payton's photo next to it. Even though I was only seven when we left Chi-town, I remember watching number 34 single-handedly take on eleven mean mofos every Sunday. Talk about battling adverse conditions and rough handling. The Bears weren't any good until they went to, and won, the Super Bowl in 1985, a decade into his pro career. He was the closest I've ever seen to a one-man team. Here's what impressed me, even then: He wasn't the fastest guy . . . he was the *toughest* guy.

My big bro Stephen and I paid homage to Sweetness in our youth. Remember that electric football game we all had as kids? We wore ours out. We'd actually put on our shoulder pads and play electric football. We made up a league consisting of eight teams, including the Bears, and we always made sure that our Walter Payton was the figure with the fastest green base. You know how you'd start the game and it would buzz and vibrate? Well, we instituted the Walter Payton rule. Whoever got Walter was allowed to stop the game, shut the power, and turn Walter once before resuming play. Hey, we were making the game more real because it meant you *couldn't* bring him down. We kept live stats, and Payton would average over 230 yards rushing per game. My parents still have the game—even though it no longer works. It's the one thing from our youth we haven't let Mom throw out.

I don't know that the meaning of Sweetness dawned on me when Stephen and I were in our shoulder pads and electrically running Payton wild back then, but I get it now: Number 34 was giving me a weekly lesson in how to stare adversity in its face. He refused to run out-of-bounds—if you were going to stop him, you had to take him down. His motto was "Never die easy," later the title of his book.

As an adult, I've bonded with others in the sports world over our hero worship of Payton. Former Steelers running back Merril Hoge is a good friend of mine. We hosted a show together, *Edge NFL Matchup*, and he played a couple of games with me in that nine-on-nine full-contact flag-football league in Waterbury, Connecticut. Merril's my age and also grew up a Payton fan. Early in his career as a running back for the Pittsburgh Steelers, he approached Payton before a game against the Bears. He was so nervous, he was practically stuttering when he said: "Excuse me, Mr. Payton, I was wondering if I could just shake your hand—I'm a big fan of yours."

"Come see me after the game," Payton said.

The Bears, just a few years removed from their dominant Super Bowl season, destroyed the Steelers in the game. Afterward, Merril found his idol at midfield. Payton, seeing his young opponent, started removing his gear—wristbands, elbow pads—and signing them for Hoge. Merril's dad was above the tunnel in the stands and took a photo of the Steelers walking through the tunnel after their shellacking. All the players had their heads down, their expressions grim after their whuppin'. But there was Merril, rocking a big ol' grin, hands held high, showing off all of Walter's stuff.

In 2003, Merril was diagnosed with stage 2 non-Hodgkins lymphoma. It was clear he took the same lesson I did from Payton's example. "It is beatable," Merril said at the time. "You have everything in you to do it. The mind is a powerful thing. There is no doubt, come May, I'll be cancer-free. Five years after that, I'll be cured. Fifty years or whatever time I have left after that, it will be the platform I stand for. I'll be a better man. This has been a blessing." Today, he is cancer-free.

In addition to Payton, my other hero was Ali. I just revered him for his resilience. Wallace D. Muhammad, the brother of Ali's manager, Herbert Muhammad, married a childhood friend of my mom's. They lived down the street from my cousins, Anthony and David (who were actually more like brothers to me). One time, when I was about six, the champ visited our neighborhood. I remember putting my fist up against his. Wow.

I knew his story early on. To me, he was a poet, an artist, and a performer, but also the baddest man on the planet. You want to talk toughness? How about the rope-a-dope? Who would come up with a strategy that has him getting thumped by the biggest blows of the baddest punchers in history—including George Foreman—only to turn the tables on his opponents once they tired themselves out? The toughest dawg out there, that's who. He decided to take the worst punishment these assassins could dish out, convinced that it would only make him stronger in the end—one of the most courageous things I'd ever seen.

But it paled in comparison to the fact that he sacrificed three years of his career in his prime and faced going to jail to stand up for what he believed in. To stand up for peace. I was too young to know or grasp all the details, but I knew that it took the ultimate in guts to do what Ali did. Talk about being alone and staring down the odds. Everybody was against him.

That resonated with me at the youngest of ages because it reminded me of my dad. Standing up for what you believed in—being principled—is what my dad was all about. Whenever I heard Ali talk, I heard the virtues and values that my dad spoke of *and* embodied.

In the epic Ali–Frazier showdowns, I was an Ali guy through and through, but I've also gotta give props to Smokin' Joe, a serious tough guy in his own right. During their legendary first fight—won by Frazier in fifteen grueling rounds—the two warriors were slugging it out in the center of the ring when Ali, always looking for an edge, tried to get inside his rival's head.

"I'm God, Joe Frazier," he taunted, throwing jabs. "You can't beat me. I'm God."

Frazier bobbed and weaved, before rising up with a counterpunch in reply. "Well, God," he said as he let loose a combination of blows. "You in the wrong place tonight."

I can't say that, in the days leading up to and following my first cancer surgery, I consciously thought of all these influences—Payton's toughness, Ali's principled stand, Frazier's doggedness—but I suspect that resilience is at least in part a learned trait. You get tough by seeing toughness in others. And I needed to get tough right quick. I didn't have a choice. I was telling my girls we were going to face this head-on. As Payton and Ali had done for me, I needed to model toughness for them.

After the surgery, I was still groggy when Dr. Milsom arrived. He was direct and to the point, which I appreciated. He'd cut me open from my chest to just above my belly button, leaving behind a big ol' twelve-inch scar. "We took out part of your large intestine and some lymph nodes," he said. "The large intestine was not cancerous. We took out twenty-eight lymph nodes. The nine that were closest to the appendix had cancer. We got all the cancer that we saw." There was no sign that the cancer had spread to the colon, kidneys, or lungs. He didn't tell me what stage I had or what the prognosis was. I didn't ask.

Instead, we talked plan of attack. Cancer cells start microscopically, he explained. In case there were some bad cells he hadn't seen, he wanted me to start a six-month round of chemotherapy once I had healed. It was late November. I targeted late December for my return to ESPN, after which I'd start chemo. Dr. Milsom shook my hand and turned to go. I was about to be alone. I was nervous. I was afraid. But I thought: *Here we go.*

WHEN I FIRST GOT DIAGNOSED, just about every executive at ESPN went out of their way to tell me the same thing: *We got you.* You wouldn't know these guys just from watching ESPN, but, more so than the talent, they're the reason the network has become as big as it is. And yet they're all so grounded. To a man, the suits—George Bodenheimer, John Skipper, John Wildhack, Mark Gross, Norby Williamson—all told me the same thing: "You take care of this first. Your job will be waiting for you."

Typical of those guys—*they* always put me first. I couldn't wait to get back to work, though, because I didn't want to sit at home doing nothing but worrying about being sick. I was scheduled to be the studio host for the Christmas Day game between the Lakers and the Suns (Kobe versus Steve Nash), but I wanted to make my first return on *SportsCenter. That* was home. I asked if I could, and my bosses were more than happy to have me anchor on December 23.

Even though I wanted to be back on-air, the truth is I was nervous about returning to the ESPN newsroom. I'd received an outpouring of support, and I was touched by all the well-wishers. But only a month into this fight, I was already experiencing what I'd come to call the Burden. There's not any time of any day that you forget you have cancer. You never have a moment when you say to yourself, *Hey, wow, I forgot I have cancer.*

That's exhausting, man. It becomes part of your identity, and it only adds to your fatigue to have the same conversation about it over and over again throughout every day. I had so many people at ESPN coming up to me saying, "Hey, how are you doing?" I hated it—which doesn't mean I didn't appreciate them. They meant well. But this cancer thing was on my mind every minute of the day—I wasn't looking to *talk* about it all day, too.

One day, late in the afternoon, I'd had enough of the parade. One guy came into my office and said, "Hey, man, how you doing?"

I'm a big believer in speaking my truth. Always have been—having cancer has only underscored for me how healthy it is to be filter-free. Plus, I was fed up. "Let me ask you something, man," I said to this well-meaning colleague. "How come this is, like, the first time you've ever been in my office?"

There was some stunned silence and an abrupt about-face. Like I said, I know I was rude. But the dude had never been in my office before. Why was he starting to care now?

One former colleague and I had some deep talks about this very subject. Robin Roberts, who had left ESPN two years before to cohost *Good Morning America*, was diagnosed with breast cancer around the same time as I got my diagnosis. She was starting six months of chemo and radiation around the same time that I'd be undergoing chemo. We were there for each other. I remember hearing about her mama's homespun wisdom long before Robin used her mama's quote for the title of her terrific book: *Everybody's Got Something*.

Robin and I would talk about how those who weren't in CancerWorld didn't get it. "Yeah," I remember Robin saying, "everyone wants to know how you're doing, and they don't get that you'll reach out to the people you want to reach out to."

The simple truth is that there's no way you can adequately respond to everyone who asks after you. First of all, there's the issue of time: If I got back to everyone who called or texted or stopped by, I wouldn't have any time left in my day. More important, though: That all takes energy, man. And it takes an expenditure of energy about something that is *already* consuming you night and day.

Robin and I used to bond over the dumb things people say to cancer patients. Our favorite was "Oh, you'll be fine! You'll beat it!" You can't believe how many people say that to you. How do *you* know I'll be fine? Where'd that medical degree of yours come from? If my oncologist can't tell me that, how can you? Others tell you about their aunt or cousin who had a similar type of cancer—and only lasted a couple of years. Thanks for sharing.

Then there are the advice-givers. The ones who tell you not to work out, what to eat. There are people who look real closely at my hairline before asking: "Have you lost any hair?" Seriously?

I know people mean well, so I feel guilty talking about them this way—but this *is* what it's like from the patient's point of view. A lot of times, people—again, meaning well—will say, "Let me know if there's anything I can do." Ummm . . . no. I'm not going to let you know if there's anything you can do. Think of the psychology of that. It's kinda putting another burden on me, man. Don't ask me what to do. Just do it. Show up at night and bring some food over. Show up during chemo and just be present. Don't overstay your welcome.

I'm close friends with my ESPN colleague Sage Steele and her husband, Jonathan. He's kind of introverted, like me, so at parties we tend to find each other in the corners of crowded rooms. One time, Sage and I were at the National Association of Black Journalists convention. At the hotel bar, a couple of guys were hitting on her.

"Hey, man," I said. "Back off."

"What do you care?" one of them said.

"She's married."

"I don't see her husband," the guy said.

"He's one of my boys," I said. "Back off." Sage seemed to appreciate me jumping in. I'm sure Jonathan appreciated it even more.

Later, after I'd started chemo, I was at the infusion center one day and Sage had said she was going to stop by. But then she texted and said, "I'm sick. Can't make it." No biggie. But there I was, sitting in that big ol' chair, all hooked up, and in walked Jonathan with biscuits. She didn't text me he was coming and he didn't ask. My man just showed up with some food. He sat there and we talked sports for a little while. When he left, there were tears in my eyes because it was such a perfect moment. All we needed was one of them awkward man hugs.

Look, not everyone can be as intuitive as Sage and Jonathan. I get that. I know people don't know what to say, so they just talk to fill the awkward silence and stuff comes out. They don't mean to say the wrong thing. But, listen, y'all: You don't have to say anything at all. Just wrap your arms around me and squeeze. A hug speaks volumes. That's what I do when I meet someone who is also in the fight. I grab on and don't let go. Or just say, "I'm really sorry you're going through this." That's all, man. It ain't hard if you keep it simple and real.

A LOT OF CANCER patients fear chemotherapy. Me, I couldn't wait to start it because I've always physically fought for something. And I wanted to show Taelor and Sydni that their dad wasn't a passive patient.

My scar from the surgery had healed. So right after New Year's, I went to the infusion center not far from my condo for my first session. This would be my routine every other Monday for at least the next twenty-four weeks. Four hours of sitting in a cushiony chair while the poison pumped into my body, followed by forty-eight hours of a chemo cocktail drip strapped to my side. Followed—immediately—by a workout at my buddy Brian's gym. And I mean *immediately.*

I can't tell you how important it felt to go from the chemo infusion center to the gym. There were patients at the infusion center who were gaunt and too weak to walk. I wanted to hug them. I wanted to work out *for* them. It took about fifteen minutes to get to the gym from the infusion center, but I felt like I was traveling a great distance: from the land of the sick to the land of the recovering. I'd work out three or four times a week, but the most important workout was the one right after chemo. It was like I was proving a point: *While you kick my butt, cancer, I'm gonna kick yours.*

That first day is when, getting on the elliptical, I noticed that name on the chemo drip. The medical name of the medicine is fluorouracil, but they call it 5-FU. That's what it said, right there: *5-FU. All right*, I thought. *A sign. FU, cancer.*

My return to the gym felt kind of spiritual. I wasn't really supposed to run since I was still connected to the port that was giving me my medicine. (Going through a port, rather than intravenously, saves the wear and tear on your veins.) I looked down, and my eye caught the logo of the manufacturer of the machine I was on: LifeStyle.

That word jumped out at me: *Life.* I started to pray, thanking God that I still had it—life. I thought back to the first thought I had when they told me in Pittsburgh: *I'm going to die.* But I was still here. And here I was, not forty-five minutes out of chemo, and I was in the gym, doing what I do. I started to run. What could be the harm? The disease wasn't in control. I was.

I skipped rope for a few minutes. Then came two sets of fifty push-ups each and a few rounds of shadowboxing. Rinse and repeat. That was followed by five sets of dumbbell bench presses—about sixty pounds each—and five sets of dumbbell curls. It wasn't one of my pre-cancer workouts, where I'd be on the treadmill for an hour and then slamming weights, but it was like medicine to me. I didn't have the girls on Mondays, but I really wanted to see them after chemo, so I'd go over to my ex-wife's house and crash in the guest bedroom. I wanted Taelor and Sydni to see me coming back from the gym, sweaty and spent, fighting for them.

I joked around with the girls about my new friend, this pack of medicine attached to my body for forty-eight hours. "He's, like, my buddy," I said. That's when we decided to name him: Marvin Fitzpatrick Bartholomew. From then on, every time they saw me after one of my post-chemo workouts, Sydni and Taelor would say hello not just to me but also to Marvin. They didn't want to be rude and ignore him.

Sydni was fascinated by the port through which "Marvin" got me my medicine. My doctor gave me a duplicate one so that

Sydni could take it to school for show-and-tell. She explained to her classmates how I got my medicine, and she told them all about her new friend Marvin.

My workouts were the most important part of my days. I hadn't done anything since the surgery, and, mentally, I needed to feel strong. I hated looking in the mirror and seeing some skinny dude with no muscle mass looking back. Maybe part of that was simple vanity, but I think it went deeper.

I'd been hardwired as an athlete since I was six years old. I thought that should give me an edge over most people who are diagnosed with cancer. I knew what it was like to work toward a physical goal, and I knew that there's no such thing as a purely physical act: the mental and physical are deeply connected.

Mentally, I needed to be in that gym. I'd talk smack to cancer like Ali talked to his opponents. A third set of push-ups? *Take that, cancer.* Twenty full-out sprint pass patterns? *Cancer, you ever run up against this?* Some kicks and punches into the middle of the heavy bag after the elliptical? *I got yer cancer right here!*

I needed to do that, not just to show my girls I was fighting for them, but also to show myself I had some control over the situation. 'Cause cancer wants to take control from you. You've got to very purposefully stand your ground. That's what going to the gym is to me. *I decide, cancer.* That's what going to work is. *I decide, cancer.* That's what traveling all over the country and abroad is. *I decide, cancer.*

I've learned as a single parent that you can't be a control freak. Man, I got teenage daughters—I've accepted not having control. I'd pick Sydni up from school at four o'clock, and her best friend, Emma, would be with her. "Dad, can Emma come over?" I love

Emma. Of course, they'd already be in the backseat by the time she asked.

"Sure," I'd say. "Of course she can." I might have had plans. But there's no such thing as planning when it comes to the life of a teenage girl. Unless Sydni had done something wrong or disrespectful, I'd never say no to her having a friend over: It's her home, too. I'd just smile and admit to myself, *I'm not really running this*. It's kind of cool. It makes every day an adventure: When you have teenage girls, you're just waiting to see what happens.

But there are some things you have to fight for control over. Remember how I used to stand over my sleeping girls late at night and vow to protect them? Cancer came into my life as a threat to them. I couldn't let it get the upper hand. Funny, as hard as I thought the fight was going to be, in subsequent years I'd learn that it's even harder. Because cancer is one formidable opponent. But so am I.

When people would hear of my post-chemo workout regimen, they'd get wide-eyed and kind of marvel at it. It's nothing to admire, folks. It's not some act of bravery. I was at the gym because I needed to be. Because I was terrified. Every minute of every day I was afraid I was going to die. Not that moment, but soon—and sooner than I'd ever thought.

You've heard the phrase *Listen to your body*? Well, during and after chemo, there were many times when I was fatigued. I wasn't nauseated so much as I just had a general *blech* feeling, a malaise. The worst feeling came three or four days after the chemo: My body felt depleted. My body seemed to be telling me to skip the gym and go home and get in bed.

I told that part of me to shut the hell up. I wasn't about to be fooled: That was the cancer talking. I'd tell myself that once I was on the elliptical, I'd start to rally. Once I shadowboxed some left-right-left combinations, the old adrenaline would kick in. Afterward, I'd crash. I wouldn't be bone-crushingly tired, but I'd be spent. If I wasn't over at Kim's to be with the girls, I'd lie on the floor in the living room at the condo while nibbling on a bland dinner and watching TV.

I'd lie there, letting my batteries recharge. One thing I've learned is that, when so much of your energy is devoted to the fight of your life, you've got to conserve energy elsewhere. On a day that I have nothing to do, I'll just lie around. That's medicine to me. There's peace of mind in being able to do that.

You even get adamant about following whatever feels right for your soul at any given moment—plans be damned. Once, I had an appointment to pee in a cup at my urologist's office. Just another in a long series of tests. Only my bladder wasn't full and it was a 78-degree, sunny day. I was faced with a choice: Do I go, and sit around for ninety minutes just so I can pee? Uh, no. It was gorgeous out. I called the doctor's office, rescheduled, and hit the golf course.

I hit balls in the blinding sunshine—and I felt so alive. My spirit felt free and warm and at peace. I felt so far away from cancer. I knew my soul needed this feeling more than another visit to another doctor's office. Calling that audible was the most empowering thing I could have done.

Cancer forces you to be selfish with your time—and you have to learn how to do that guilt-free. A lot of times, when I need to go from Bristol to New York City, I'll call a limo service. The girls get on me and tell me I'm rude because, when the driver starts to chitchat with me, I'll just say: "Hey, man, I don't want to talk."

That's not rude, I'll tell them. It's direct. "You'll hurt his feelings," they say. I can't be responsible for his feelings. This cancer stuff is heavy, man. When Taelor talks to me about going to grad school, I don't say it aloud, but what I'm thinking is *Will I be here for that?* That's a lot to deal with. I can't add the limo driver's feelings to my list of concerns. Or the friend who invited me over whom I've called at the last minute to say I can't make it. I might not have a good reason; I just don't feel up to it. I know to avoid being somewhere where my spirit isn't going to feel good. If that ticks off my friend, how good a friend is he or she? I can't think about how someone else feels about it. That's their problem to handle. I got this problem over here, and it's a mutha.

I think our society is too concerned with how other people feel. When a guy accidentally bumps into you, what's your natural reaction? You say, "Oh, I'm sorry, excuse me." Why are you apologizing? *He* just bumped into *you!* You don't want him to feel bad. But you're not responsible for his feelings.

I want to be clear. I'm not saying you're in this fight alone. I'm just saying you have a responsibility *to* the fight. If I'm too exhausted to call somebody back and they call again and say, "Hey, you didn't call me back," I say, simply: "Yeah." I couldn't, man. And I'm not going to feel bad about that.

Here's the way I look at it. Remember during the coverage of Hurricane Katrina, those images of people on their roofs while makeshift boats full of people sailed by? Well, this is my boat-people analogy. We've been flooded and I'm in a boat that's gliding by everyone I know on top of those roofs. But my boat only holds fifteen people. I got my girls, my family, my closest friends. When your boat is full, it's not like you're saying to everyone else on those roofs, "I don't care about you." It's just that these are my boat people and I've gotta save *them*.

Because they're in the fight with me. This is crucial: When you take on cancer, you're *not* alone. Of course, that's not how it feels when you first hear those words: "You have cancer." At that moment, you feel more alone than you've ever been. You're standing in place, numb, and the world is rushing by.

But then you start to realize that others stand with you.

There's the cancer-fighting community, which is strong and tight. When I meet someone with cancer, we have an instant bond. We hug tight and we talk in clipped shorthand.

"I'm five years in," he or she will say.

"Two months," I'd reply. Sometimes I'd say, "Newbie," like: Show me the ropes.

The bond isn't for show. You're finally around someone who gets it. They get what it's like to sit for hours getting chemo pumped into your body. They get what it's like to have people look at you with that pained expression on their face and whisper, "So how *are* you?" They get what it's like to constantly have to go to the bathroom. They get what it's like to have taking a crap become such a big part of your life. They get what it's like to never have a run-of-the-mill stomachache again, because every little cramp, pain, and twinge triggers the thought: *Is that cancer?* You don't even have to discuss these things. It's just a relief knowing there's someone who has been where you've been.

Robin Roberts was one of those people for me. We had both

spent the previous six months undergoing chemo when together we presented the 2008 Jimmy V Perseverance Award to Bills tight end Kevin Everett at the ESPYs—the first time it was held at LA's Nokia Theatre. Everett had miraculously overcome paralysis suffered during a kickoff collision. When Robin and I walked out, I in a dark suit with an open collar, she stylin' in a striking blue dress, we were greeted with loud applause.

"This year," I said, "the 2008 ESPY Celebrity Golf Classic raised over $1 million for the Jimmy V Foundation, with all proceeds—every single penny—going directly to cancer research. And this past year, both Robin and I—" I nodded toward her, and she to me—"discovered personally that fighting cancer is something we can never give up on."

"In fact," Robin said, "it was exactly a year ago that I was diagnosed with breast cancer, and I was comforted by the memory of being there that night at the ESPYs when Jimmy V said those powerful words: 'Don't give up. Don't ever give up.' He inspired a whole generation of coaches and athletes and taught them what it takes to truly be a winner."

Robin is just all class. Funny, most times when we've bonded over our cancer battles, they haven't been real long conversations. You don't need to have a long talk. It's just: "How is it for you?" followed by a hug or a fist bump. Maybe a "hang in there."

But it means the world. Because she's been there. She gets it. Same with Lance Armstrong, who sent me an e-mail from Africa, where he was on a goodwill tour, shortly after I was diagnosed. "I'm here, man," he wrote. "If you ever want to talk, ever want some advice about anything."

I didn't ask for any advice, just thanked him, told him how

much I appreciated his reaching out. Every few months after that exchange, I'd get an e-mail from him, just checking in. "How's it going? Hang in there," he'd write. That mattered, man. It might seem like a cliché, but it mattered—because of who he is. This guy had brain cancer and cancer in his testicles. He was supposed to die, and he came off the table and won seven Tour de France titles. I know, I know, he cheated on the bike. Okay, but every one of his opponents was probably also juiced up. And I don't really care about a bike race. I draw inspiration from the kind of cancer fighter he was. He did it, and now he was telling me I could do it, too.

One day, I got a call from Ernie Johnson of TNT. I had met him maybe once. But he had battled cancer in his past, and he must have checked in with me three or four times after that. The first time we talked, we were on the phone for an hour. Man, dudes don't talk on the phone for an hour about anything, but there we were, swapping cancer tales. I'll never forget that. He made me feel like I was part of a team.

Then there was my cancer-fighting community closer to home. My friend Barb had had loved ones in the fight and knew before I did that I was going to have to learn to be strategic with my supply of energy. So without telling me, she hired an assistant for me, so that I'd have someone who could pick up my dry cleaning, go grocery shopping, and pay my bills.

And there were friends like Laura Okmin, the Fox Sports reporter, whose mom had cancer. I'd never met her mother, but from what Laura told me, her mother was one of those people with a personality that lit up a room—even going through cancer and chemo. Laura shared with me how close her mom's on-cologist had grown to her mom—and how rare that was. When her mom passed away, the doctor was at the funeral. That's when Laura explained to me that oncologists usually had to protect themselves from getting so close. It helped me realize that I need my doctors for their expertise and that I had people like Laura, my family, and other close friends for love and support.

Also in my dugout is Deedee Mills. I first met Deedee fifteen years ago when she worked in the Carolina Panthers' front office. She left the Panthers, adopted an adorable six-year-old Ethiopian boy, Cannon (to him, I'm "Uncle Stuart"), which prompted her to start the Behailu Academy, an after-school arts program for underprivileged kids. She's also a cancer survivor. Whenever I'm struggling with a decision—settling on a course of treatment, let's say—she'll ask a series of questions until it becomes apparent to me what I should do. She has a skill for taking me down this road where the answer is obvious at the end. "You know what to do," she'll say.

Then there's Amy Bartlett. She works for Nike, managing its relationship with Tiger Woods. I'd known her casually, chatting with her at some Tiger Woods Foundation events. But when I was first diagnosed, a mutual friend told me she was a cancer survivor and that I should talk to her. I gave her a call and opened the conversation with: "I hear you know a little something about what I'm going through." From then on, we just clicked.

Amy has a talent for reaching out right when I need it the most. I'll get a text from her that reads: "Hey. No need to re-spond. Played golf today and was just thinking about you." I'll text back: "Hope you broke 90." It was her way of checking in to see how I was doing—without talking about cancer. We'd use golf as therapy.

A couple of years ago, on the five-year anniversary of her remission, she climbed Mount Kilimanjaro with other cancer survivors as part of a Livestrong cancer research fund-raiser. At the top, she planted an honor flag with my name on it. After that, another one of my boys—former Livestrong CEO Doug Ulman—also climbed Kilimanjaro, and *he* planted an honor flag in my name. "You've got to be the only guy to have had *two* flags up there!" Amy told me.

Doug and I have some deep conversations; he's always telling me I don't understand the impact I have on others. I hear that, but I'm not comfortable with it, for the same reason I'm not comfortable when I hear myself described as "courageous." 'Cause I know what I really feel. And I feel afraid, not brave.

I have a small group of close guy friends, and we don't talk like other guys talk. With Doug and my boys Brian Gallagher and Dr. Scott Organ—Scottie—we get into it, man. Sure, there's a lot of golf and a lot of working out. But there are also a lot of late-night, soul-searching phone conversations—the kind of deep *What does it all mean?* bull sessions too many of us last had back in our college dorm-room days.

Yeah, when people ask me how I get up and attack cancer every day, there are two answers: What choice do I have? And: These people, man. These are my boat people.

CHAPTER NINE

NOW WHAT?

The last time the Lakers and Celtics met in the NBA Finals, I was debating whether to take a $200-per-week job in Florence, South Carolina. I remember watching Magic Johnson's baby hook shot silence Larry Bird's Celtics while I was agonizing over whether to go to work at WPDE. I called around, seeking advice, thinking that this would be the most important decision of my life.

What's that line? Don't sweat the small stuff—and it's all small stuff. Now it was twenty-one years later, and as I was getting ready to cover a series between Kobe Bryant's Lakers and Kevin Garnett's Celtics, I was learning that, while it's not *all* small stuff, most things aren't as big as you thought when you look at them through the rearview mirror. That's something cancer does for you: It smacks you in the face with instant perspective.

In another month, Robin and I would present the Jimmy V Perseverance Award at the ESPYs. But first, in June 2008, came those NBA Finals and a personal milestone: my last scheduled chemotherapy sessions.

When the Finals began, I underwent what was to be my next-to-last session—followed, of course, by a trip to the gym. A couple of days later, I went to the hospital for a scan. By now I had learned more about the art of detecting cancer than I'd ever wanted to know. It is, at least partly, an art, because cancer doesn't want you to find it. There are many ways to discover cancer: X-ray, MRI, CT scan, and PET-CT scan, which tends to give you more 3-D angles and images. But here's the tricky part: Some tumors might show up better on, say, a CT scan than on a PET-CT scan. Some tumors hide behind organs or look like blockages or scar tissue.

The kind of cancer I'd been diagnosed with was especially hard to detect. To do so, doctors need a baseline set of scans for comparison purposes. They had my scans from when I was first diagnosed six months before, and now they'd compare those to this one and other scans that awaited in the future.

When they slide you into the PET machine, your arms stretched out above your head, it's like sliding into a close, tight tunnel. I get claustrophobic, so I shut my eyes before they pushed me back into the big, humming machine. Once in, I heard the engine gear up and start to whir, followed by a disembodied voice instructing me to hold my breath and then exhale, over and over again. Thirty minutes later, I was taking off that flimsy robe and getting dressed, my sights set on the upcoming Game One of the Lakers–Celtics throw-down.

At that game, I ran into Mike Breen. I'd known him for years, but never all that well. The TV play-by-play man for the Finals, Breen is around my age and a New York guy through and through. He was the voice of the New York Knicks, lived out on Long Island, had gone to Fordham. He's a quiet, reserved guy who I'd always thought of as a pro's pro. And, like me, he loved nothing better than to hit the links on a sunny day when he had a few hours. In the media room before Game One of the Finals, we compared notes on our golf games and agreed to find a Bean-town course together the next day.

The details of our day on the links are fuzzy to me now. I have no idea what I shot or what Breen shot. I don't remember what hole we were on when my cell phone rang. I just remember what the voice on the other end of the line had to say.

"Stuart, this is Dr. Jeffrey Baker," he said. My oncologist at Hartford Hospital. I walked over to a nearby veranda for privacy.

"I've been over your scan and wanted to give you a call," he said. "I don't see any signs of cancer."

There was silence.

"Well," I said, finally. "What does this mean?"

"Cancerous cells aren't showing up on your scan anymore," he said. In case I wasn't getting it, he added: "This is a good thing."

I was quiet. He filled the silence. "There are no masses, no chunks of anything," he said. "This is a good thing."

Had he used the word "remission" I would have been skeptical. I'd learned to hate the language typically used in Cancer-World. For example, the phrase "cancer survivor" normally applied to someone who has "beaten" cancer with five years of clean scans. That's crazy stupid. If you're living with a diagnosis of cancer and you wake up the next morning, you should then and there be considered a cancer survivor—period. Every day you've survived cancer. Every day is a win.

My whole professional life revolved around reporting wins and losses, so you'd think I'd be comfortable with the idea that cancer is something that you either "beat" or "lose to." But the more time I spent in CancerWorld, the more I was struck by these simplistic ways we talk about it. As I listened to the stories of my fellow cancer fighters at the infusion center, to their tales about how cancer hides and jukes and feints you, how it can lull you into a false sense of security, I realized that *how* we think and talk about cancer is part of the problem.

I vowed never to use words like "remission" or phrases like "beat cancer." Maybe it had to do with never wanting to let my guard down. In boxing, they say the punches most likely to knock you out are those you don't see coming. I never wanted to *not* see cancer coming again—I'd rather brace myself for the blow.

"Does this mean I don't have cancer anymore?" I asked the doc.

Dr. Baker paused, choosing his words carefully. When I first started seeing him, I was put off by how distant Dr. Baker could be. But that's when my friend, Laura Okmin—one of my boat people—explained to me that oncologists often *have* to be cold and clinical out of self-protection. So many of their patients don't make it—they can't allow themselves to get emotionally invested. Once I heard that, I was able to focus on Dr. Baker's expertise and not his demeanor, which was always professional, if not overly warm. And that combination of personality traits wasn't unique to him. As Laura had predicted, my other oncologist, Dr. Manish Shah at New York–Presbyterian, was also one cool customer.

Here's where I truly appreciated Dr. Baker's "just the facts" demeanor. I needed to make sense of what he was telling me, and he was giving it to me straight. "It means there's no cancer we can detect," he said. "I want to consult with the rest of your team, but I think we should skip your last chemotherapy, and then we'll get you on a schedule of a scan every six months. If, after five years, those are all clean, we can go to a scan once a year. Sound good?"

What the hell. I should have been ecstatic, I know. But I wasn't feeling anything. I felt like I'd entered another world. I wasn't grounded. I was floating—that's all I remember. The sensation of floating. I dialed my dad's number, but I got his voice mail. Hung up.

I just sat there and took some deep breaths. The sun beat down on my face; the air filled my lungs. It was quiet. I looked around at the expanse of green before me—trees and fairway, as far as I could see. *How blessed I am to be out here*, I thought, basking in the silence, the sun, the view. Just then, Breen walked up.

"Hey, man," I said softly, "that was my doctor. I don't have to do any more chemo. They couldn't find any cancer in my latest scan."

I said this almost like a question—as if I were asking if it could be true. It felt weird to hear the words leaving my mouth.

I don't remember what Mike Breen said, but it was entirely appropriate for the situation and our relationship. He was happy for me, but we were subdued. There were no high-fives or end-zone-like gyrations. Poor guy. He'd wanted a little afternoon escape and now he found himself in some all-too-real drama. But he handled it like the pro he's always been. Later, that day would form a bond between us. Whenever we were in a big group of media types at the Finals or All-Star Weekend, I'd say, "This is the first man I told when I learned I had my first clean scan," and we'd nod at each other.

But that day, I don't recall if I was even fully aware of Breen's presence. Even in the car after our round, I felt foggy and dis-jointed. It was only later, hours later, that it hit me. And it wasn't a feeling of relief that hit me, like you'd think. No, it was a feeling of anxiety. Two words occurred to me, and they kept bouncing around my brain:

Now what?

A COUPLE OF YEARS AGO, a study of cancer patients showed something very interesting. Two years after a cancer diagnosis, the average level of depression among patients tends to drop back down to match the general population. But after completing a course of cancer treatment, the level of *anxiety* among patients booms.

I totally get it. One day, you're in the fight: Your calendar is filled with scans, blood work, biopsies, and doctor's appointments. You hang on your doctor's every word. Then—just like that—you hear that it's gone, that "there are no visible signs of cancer" in your body, and you're as mentally unprepared for that as you were when you first got your diagnosis.

Don't get me wrong. Being in the fight sucked. Going to chemo once every two weeks, dealing with its aftereffects, living in CancerWorld—all of it sucked. But at least you were in the fight. Once you're told your cancer is gone, so is the thing you've made your single focus every day.

Now what?

I'd seen it in sports: Once your nemesis is gone, you feel a letdown. When Björn Borg retired, Johnny Mac went into a funk. Frazier was so set on chasing Ali to the ends of the earth that he lost to big George Foreman. I should have been jubilant, I know. But I couldn't wrap my head around what could be next. I'd been this warrior cancer guy. "Cancer fighter" had become the way I thought of myself.

Now, suddenly, I was being told I wasn't who I thought I was. What hits home at a moment like that is just how much you are forever changed once you have cancer. A study released by the Duke Cancer Center in 2011 found that four out of ten cancer patients are plagued by symptoms of post-traumatic stress disorder for as long as a decade after the end of their treatment. It was like having been to war: flashbacks, depression, anxiety. I felt it every day. Cancer robs you of the ability to grow old, to have the same aches and pains of aging that your contemporaries experience. My buddy Brian wakes up feeling sore in the morning and thinks, *Man, this getting-old thing is a pain.* I wake up feeling sore and think, *Is that cancer? Is it back?*

That anxiety never leaves you. In fact, it only gets worse—because you're no longer taking proactive steps to combat the disease. I guess that's what this really comes down to: Like so many patients, I didn't believe that my cancer was gone, not really. I'd learned what a worthy opponent cancer was. I was scared it was rope-a-doping me.

That's why, in the days following the news from Dr. Baker, I felt like I'd been sent out to fight without live ammo, like I was now cut loose from my support and would be shooting blanks against cancer from now on. I know, I know: You're probably thinking, *C'mon, dude, can't you just accept good news for what it is?*

I understand the logic of that reaction, but I gotta tell you: I know from talking to other patients, it just doesn't work that way. You want me to stop worrying now? I've done nothing *but* worry since the day of my diagnosis. Add to that how hard it is to detect rogue appendiceal cancer cells, and that my type of cancer doesn't really go into true, all-out remission, and you have a recipe for more anxiety, not less.

Once, when I was a few years into the fight, I asked Lance Armstrong if he still thought about cancer—and dying from it—every single day. "No, not anymore," he said.

And how long did it take him to get to the point that it wasn't on his mind daily?

He smiled. "About twelve years," he said. "It took me a while."

It took a lot for me to ask Lance that question. I know they say you should ask a lot of questions as a cancer patient, but sometimes I found just the opposite. I started to avoid asking questions if I thought the answers to them could make me more worried and scared. Had Lance said, "Oh, the minute I had a clean scan, I put cancer behind me," I would have obsessed over what was wrong with me: Why couldn't I do the same?

Instead, Lance's example was one of many that proved to me how complicated it is to live with cancer now as a part of your biography.

IN MAY 2008 I went in for the first of my six-month scans. It was a stat PET-CT scan. If you remember early episodes of the TV show *ER*, you remember a young doctor who would later become George Clooney yelling at a young nurse who would later become Julianna Margulies something like: "The patient's heart just stopped! We need a defibrillator in here *stat*!"

In medical lingo, "stat" means immediately. I was scheduled to get immediate results. The radiologist would call my oncologist, who would call me right after the test, often before I got home. On the one hand, this meant there would be no sleepless nights spent wondering if the cancer had returned. But it also meant that the anxiety was now front-loaded. On my way to the hospital, I steeled myself for hearing the words "Your cancer has returned."

Once the scan was over, I reminded the nurse that this was a stat scan. I had just reached my car when Dr. Baker called.

"We don't see anything," he said.

And so it went. A succession of clean stat scans followed: November 2008. May 2009. November 2009.

Still, I wasn't satisfied. I kept wondering, *When's it going to come back?* When I was fighting cancer—doing chemo, kicking its butt in the gym—at least I felt like I was taking back some control from the disease. Even though I was still doing my thing in the gym and had gotten into the craziness that is mixed martial arts, the wait now between scans was long and hard. It felt like I was being passive—something I promised I'd never be. In January 2010, I went to see Dr. Milsom, my surgeon. I told him I wanted to do something. "Is there some preventative chemo I could take? Or can we go in arthroscopically to see if anything is happening in there?" I asked.

I prevailed upon him to go in and take a look. There was nothing there besides the scar tissue that had formed after my last surgery. He scraped it away.

I'm a positive person—the way I'd stared down cancer in the first place should show that—but despite the scans and Dr. Milsom's findings, I kept wondering, *Is the cancer back?* I was hyper-aware of my body. The simplest twinge or gas bubble set off alarms. I even did a round of preventative chemo. I wanted to make sure I was doing everything I could to avoid it coming back.

Then came November 2010. After the scan, getting into my car, my phone rang. "Stuart, it's Dr. Baker," he said. He knew me well enough by now to dispense with the small talk. "It's another clean scan," he said. "I see no signs of cancer cells." Keep it up, he said.

Nine days later, I took Taelor and Sydni to a matinee showing of *A Christmas Carol* at the Hartford Stage, a great theater in Hartford, Connecticut. A buddy of mine from junior high school was the stage director. I was thrilled to be there with my girls, but halfway through the performance I started to worry that *I* was being visited by the ghost of cancers past. I had a bad stom-achache, and that set off the alarms. *It was only nine days since a clean scan, so it couldn't be cancer, right? Or could it be?*

When the pain wouldn't subside, I called my doctors. Tests were ordered. An endoscopy. An ultrasound. "I don't see any-thing definitive," Dr. Milsom said. "But this area right here"—he pointed—"looks a little cloudy. That doesn't look right. I'd like to go in and take a look."

So we planned it for right after the holidays and New Year's. I was dating a woman who was a professional dancer. She and her troupe were performing New Year's Eve at a party on the rooftop of a hotel in Tampa, Florida. She asked if I wanted to be in it. I could do a waltz, and if I was feeling confident, I could also dance in one of their hip-hop routines. Bring on the hip-hop. I handled my business that night.

Afterward, it felt like another descent into CancerWorld. I was now a veteran and had learned how to decode things. This felt different from the procedure Dr. Milsom performed in January. Before surgery, the anesthesiologist asked if I should be given an epidural. In early 2010, Dr. Milsom's answer to that question was "Not necessary." Now it was "Yeah, let's go ahead, just in case."

Before I went under, I remember thinking, *Uh-oh. Not a good sign.* When I woke up, I learned that Dr. Milsom had removed three big tumors and a lot of scar tissue. He went in through the same twelve-inch scar as before. He took out part of the small intestine and part of the colon.

I was back in the fight.

CHAPTER TEN

BACK IN
THE RING

learned that courage was not the absence of fear, but the triumph over it," Nelson Mandela once said. "The brave man is not he who does not feel afraid, but he who conquers that fear."

Amen, brotha. Talk about resilient dudes. I never got to meet Mandela, but early in my career I covered a speech he gave in Atlanta on his first trip to the States after he was released from prison—after twenty-seven years. Think about that: twenty-seven years behind bars for your beliefs. I remember watching him that day and thinking, *This is one tough ol' dude.* You didn't want to step to him in the street. No surprise that he'd been a boxer. He could take a punch.

After my surgery, I had to do what Mandela was talking about. I had to look my fear in the face. I had plenty of time to think. I got an infection and was in the hospital for fourteen days. I had wanted to be back and healthy for the Super Bowl, Giants versus Patriots, Eli versus Tom Terrific, but now I'd be lucky just to be back home where I could watch it on my hi-def flat-screen. I was so down and so scared that I called the wisest person I know, my big sister Susan. And I told her: "You're going to have to start working on my eulogy."

And this is one of the ways Susan is so wise. She didn't say,

"Oh, c'mon, you'll be okay." She didn't panic. She didn't try to talk me out of my feelings. She didn't give me a pep talk. Instead she said, "Let me get this straight—you want to talk about something that is probably not going to happen until you are ninety and I'm ninety-seven? Okay, if that's what you need me to do." She knew this was a process and, right now, I was facing something and needed to work my way through it.

Fear's an interesting thing. I come from the macho world of sports. Growing up, we're taught to not be afraid. But now I was learning what that whole mind-set was really about—denial. I was learning it's okay to be afraid. It's okay to be afraid of dying. This idea of be brave, don't cry, get over it—whatever the phrase is—was bull. I'm so glad I was raised in a family where crying was never seen as showing weakness. Having emotions is healthy. Fear is normal.

Look, it's complicated. Our culture tells us not to give in to fear, to be brave. I totally believe that. That's why the Mandela quote resonates with me. That's why I would keep going to the gym, keep fighting. But it's not totally black-and-white. Sometimes it's smart to listen to your fear. Once, I had the opportunity to fly with the Blue Angels, the Navy flight show. No, thank you, not this brotha. I passed on it and I don't mind telling you why: I was afraid. Now, part of that had to do with the pressure in my eyes. If a plane went too fast, it could do me some damage. But mostly it was just this: Something could go wrong. I didn't want to take that chance.

My boys were, like, "Man, you scared."

I was, like, "Damn right I'm scared."

See, I believe in looking straight at your fear—but that doesn't mean you *always* gotta go *mano a mano* against it. And you should never, ever feel like you're "less than" if you don't do something because you're afraid. Man, you got cancer: You *should* be afraid, and that *should* change your calculations. But you also should never stop dealing with it—which is what Mandela was getting at.

Knowing that my cancer was back—though, in reality, it probably had never left and was instead just undetectable—I lost some hope. But it also gave me a jolt of necessary realism. Now, when I thought back to when Dr. Baker told me in 2008 that my scan showed no signs of cancer but that some cancers were hard to see this way, I remember feeling bullheaded at the time, like, *You'll be able to see mine.* That kind of cocky confidence was now long gone. After all, these tumors were found nine days after a clean scan. From now on, I realized, *I'll never know for sure.* Now my mind-set was going to be more fatalistic as I went home to heal and then start a new round of chemo: *Okay, let's do this. And let's wait and see how long it takes to grow back again.*

I WAS DETERMINED TO acknowledge my fear, yes, but damned if I was going to do things to make it worse. I learned some lessons the first time around. I wasn't about to search the Internet for information about my disease, hoping against hope that there was some magic treatment or pill out there. I knew from last time that seemingly every cancer story on the Internet is about dying.

When you have cancer and you start scouring the Internet, you find a lot of negativity. This time, I knew enough not to want to become an expert. This time, I knew enough to do what feels good for my soul. This time, I was okay with some people thinking I wasn't as informed as I should be—because I knew it was better for my spirit to *not* be quite so informed. Rather than seeking out answers myself by going online, I'd get informed by calling my doctors and saying, "This is what's going on. What do I do about it?"

Those guys are my medical dream team. At New York–Presbyterian, Dr. Milsom is a world-class surgeon and Dr. Shah is a leading oncologist. The reserved Dr. Jeffrey Baker has impeccable credentials. And my urologist in Connecticut, Dr. Hugh Kennedy, will actually text or call for no reason, just to see how I'm doing. This even though, more than once, I've left his office without realizing that I was still clutching his waiting-room copy of *Sports Illustrated*. When I'd apologize, his receptionist would tell me to just go ahead and help myself to them.

As much as I like them and am grateful for them, I'd like to not be in constant contact with my doctors. Having a standing weekly check-in, for example, would make me feel too much like a cancer patient. I want to talk to them only when I have to. They're all very good about talking to one another—I always feel like everyone is on the same page when I make medical decisions, and that's crucial.

I could have gone another way. Friends, relatives, and even well-meaning strangers all suggested alternative treatments. One friend took his special-needs daughter to South America for a holistic cancer regimen—there's supposed to be some guru doctor down there with some answers.

I don't discard that—I'm all for whatever works for you, man.

But I felt like I had to make a choice: either go the traditional-medicine route or not. There are a lot of alternative treatments that focus on diet—some say that a third of the food you eat should be raw and that foods like broccoli should be eaten every day. The problem is, having now had my stomach resected a couple of times, I couldn't necessarily digest all those leafy things. If I ate that stuff, instead of being on the toilet seven times a day, I'd be on it *all* day.

No, now that I was back in the fight, I was doubling down on my medicine and my doctors. But first I had to recover enough to get back in the gym, back to work, and back on chemo. And that meant healing enough to lose my Wound VAC.

Even though I was home, the twelve-inch scar down my chest and abdomen, which was about three-quarters of an inch wide, wasn't closed. It looked like something out of a slasher movie. It was hooked up to this vacuum that continually sucks fluid from the wound and increases blood flow to it. I ain't gonna lie: It's kinda gross. I tried to get the girls to name the Wound VAC in the same way we named the chemo drip, but they weren't having that. This contraption wasn't cute to them, like Marvin Fitzpatrick Bartholomew had been.

A nurse would come every few days to change the dressing and make sure I was healing properly. I wasn't supposed to get the wound wet, so showers were out. I had to bathe the old-school way, standing up at the sink.

Soon I started to notice a change in the girls this time around. Taelor was now sixteen and Sydni twelve. They'd been wide-eyed and emotionally open last time around—three years ago now. They'd asked questions. Now they were more stone-faced and not as interested in talking about what I was going through. That's natural, right? I mean, they were teenagers, or, in Sydni's case, nearly a teenager . . . they're *supposed* to grow more sullen and harder to read, right?

No doubt, that was it. But I also wondered if their silence was about something else: fear. After all, it looked like I was being what I'd always said I wouldn't be: nothing but a cancer patient. I was home, all the way down to 160 pounds, and strapped to that damned Wound VAC all day.

I'd always joke with them about my toughness and physicality, and they'd roll their eyes at me—like, *Look what I have to put up with.* "Sydni, how many dads at your school you think can beat me in a race?" I'd ask.

She'd sigh. "Dad, no one cares."

"*None!* That's how many!"

Or: "Hey, Taelor, you think any of your friends' dads could last more than a round with me?"

Another sigh. "How old *are* you?" she'd ask.

But now I was wondering if they secretly wished I had that swagger back. I wondered if there was something about seeing me lying there, hooked up to that machine, literally wounded, that was messing with them. If you've ever been the dad of teenage girls, you know that when a thought like that occurs to you, it's a nonstarter to try to discuss it with them. You'll get those one-word, monotone answers, like when you ask, "What'd you do in school today?"

"Nothin'," you'll be told, in a flat, uninterested tone.

No, this wasn't about starting a conversation. It was about showing that I'm still *me*. It's about getting up off that couch, getting back in the gym, and getting better. I started to think about what it feels like to have that bounce in your step, like you're feeling strong. I started to will myself toward that feeling. Within a few weeks, the wound had closed. I was ready to get back in the ring. Literally.

LAST TIME, I WAS nervous walking back into the ESPN newsroom. This time, I dreaded it. Because I knew what waited for me there: more questions. Unending questions. And when I wasn't at work, I'd be at the gym . . . where strangers would walk up and ask how I'm doing.

I appreciated that they cared, but it sapped me. Rather than hitting Brian's gym, I started doing P90X at home. I'd started chemo again—this time, a cocktail called FOLFIRI. I'd follow it with P90X as soon as I got home from the infusion center. P90X is an intense workout developed by Tony Horton that mixes elements of yoga, Pilates, and plyometrics with upper and lower body workouts. I'd pull out a yoga mat and my weights right in my living room, pop in a P90X DVD, and get busy. The workout is less than an hour, but there's no rest. Your heart gets pumping right quick. After, I'd be wiped out and I'd just lie on the floor, recharging. I'd have dinner right there, watching TV—*Parenthood* is another favorite—and I'd treat myself to a glass of red wine.

If I wasn't doing P90X, I was over at Plus One Defense doing mixed martial arts. I'd pop in the mouthpiece that I'd inscribed with Taelor's and Sydni's initials, put on my goggles (gotta guard those eyes!), and slide on my headgear. I'd walk to the center of the gray and blue padded floor, defiant. *You thought you had me down, cancer . . . but here I am.*

I'd spar with a handful of guys, including some local cops and Darin Reisler, the gym's owner. We'd go at it, getting our jujitsu and Muay Thai on, the *thump-thump* of our punches and kicks echoing in the air. We'd work on moves, like rear naked chokeholds, triangle arm bars, and the guillotine. We'd fight in a steel cage.

Whenever I was on that mat, going at it, I felt like a warrior . . . but a peaceful warrior. And I needed to feel like that, like I was fighting back—literally and figuratively. Physical hand-to-hand combat is the ultimate test. You get revealed *and* you reveal things about yourself: who's stronger, who's trained better. But MMA training is mostly about the mind and being calm and repeating what you've been taught. You learn the type of punishment you'll withstand. You learn to deliver punishment in reply. When things go bad and you hurt, that's when you have to be at your most calm. That's when you learn that the rough patches have endings, too.

When you have cancer, all this is the best medicine for your soul. It's not so much about being the best fighter out there—it's really about being out there, period. Taking blows, delivering blows, and walking away, knowing that you left every ounce of energy on the mat. There's personal satisfaction in that—even on days you get thumped. You get it if, like me, you're someone who was born to play sports, drawn by the competition and the jolt of physical contact.

Within months, I watched myself transform. I'd look at myself in the mirror when I first got home from the hospital and I'd see a skinny dude with no muscle definition attached to a Wound VAC. Now, I was getting back to me. I could see the muscle mass returning. My cardio was back. I was starting to feel that old bounce in my step. I was up to 185 pounds. I was in the best shape I'd been in since minicamp with the Jets nine years earlier.

One day, coming back from MMA training, I stopped at Starbucks for my usual protein smoothie. I'd done P90X the day before. It was unseasonably warm and the sun contributed to my good mood. I was going to go home, rest awhile, and then do P90X again—a two-workout day. I got my smoothie and didn't so much as walk out of Starbucks as *glide*. I had a familiar feeling, like when I was sixteen and aware of my body while I walked, aware of my own strength. Oh, that feeling. You don't know what it's like to feel strong until you've been weak. *Man, I'm ripped, I'm shredded*, I told myself. *I'm strong and fit . . . and I have cancer.*

How weird that I could feel like this *and* have cancer. *That's okay*, I told myself. *I'm fit and strong. And cancer can't take that away from me.* I got in my car and headed home. P90X was waiting for me.

IN AUGUST 2011, an army invaded Philadelphia. We were an army of cancer fighters, all supporting one another on the front lines. It was the Livestrong Challenge, a weekend bike race and fund-raiser. More than five thousand cyclists and nearly one thousand volunteers came together for a weekend that raised $2.8 million for the fight.

But the thing I'll always remember is the act of coming together. I've never felt such fellowship. Everywhere you turned, you saw a teammate. Ever been surrounded by people and know that everyone you look at is with you in a common cause? It's a mind-blowing feeling.

At the end of the weekend, I was asked to share the stage with Lance Armstrong and Doug Ulman. We were under a huge tent in Valley Forge, just outside Philly, and we told our stories. Doug told moving personal stories that showed how the funds that Livestrong raises go directly to saving lives. At one point, Doug presented the top individual and team fund-raising awards, and one went to this old-timer named Dave, whose goal had been "70-70-70": He had just turned seventy, he had biked seventy miles, and his goal had been to raise $70,000—which he surpassed by $15,000. How cool is that?

Honestly, I don't remember all of what Lance, Doug, and I said. But it wasn't about what was said. It was about being there with everyone else. It hit me harder than ever before that a roomful of cancer fighters is a powerful place. Everyone there either had cancer or loved someone who had cancer.

I was dating a woman at the time whose aunt was battling pancreatic cancer. Her aunt and I had grown tight since we were going through chemo at the same time. The month before, she'd been in a real bad place, but she rallied enough to come to Philly from her small town in Florida with her boyfriend, an energetic Vietnam vet whose first wife had died of cancer. It was the first time they'd been around other people with cancer. Just being there was monumental for them. When you've been through what a cancer patient has been through, this stuff matters. Feeling like you're part of something bigger—a movement—matters.

It goes beyond just having a sense of strength in numbers. You can be around thousands of people and still feel alone if you don't feel any bond. That whole weekend, there was a feeling of camaraderie in the air. We were all fighting the same thing—it's strength in numbers, yes, but it's strength in numbers with a shared experience. We link arms and we fight.

Cancer's this big, bad fifty-foot monster and you usually feel like you're fighting this thing by yourself. I love underdogs, but it's draining to *always* be David going up against Goliath. Now there were thousands of us. This is what it felt like: *You might pick off a few of us here and there, cancer, but for this day, for this moment . . . we're going to beat you.*

I was so moved, I left a video message for all who came—and for those that couldn't make it—on the Livestrong website. I wore a Livestrong cycling jersey and spoke into the camera. "I just wanted to say thank you. This weekend, this family gathering, was so important to me . . ." I said. "I'm battling cancer for the second time, and it's a family effort. Twenty-eight million cancer survivors, their loved ones, people that care about them. We are not a small but a very large army, and we put our finances, our time, our space, our energy all together to try to rid the world of this ridiculously ugly, savage disease. . . . Because of the camaraderie and the togetherness of this entire weekend, the struggle is a lot easier. Because you always have somebody to lean on. We're all in this together. I just want to thank Livestrong for giving me the opportunity to come share, to hopefully inspire, and to be inspired by all of you."

I was already working my butt off in the fight—but now I was like a wideout bursting out of the locker room onto the field during the pregame intros. I went after it. How could I not? I left Philly that weekend knowing it's not just me. An army had my back, and I had theirs.

I continued to take on cancer the only way I knew how: by living my life to the fullest. In May 2012, my scan was clean once again. This time, the wording was a little different: "No new evidence of disease."

That fit my mind-set. I wasn't being told that there was no cancer in my body—just that there was no new evidence of cancer. That's like telling me to keep my guard up. Unlike last time, the clean scan didn't take me by surprise. I knew enough by now to know it wouldn't change my approach: *I'm still in the fight.*

NOT LONG AFTER MY latest clean scan, I was hanging with my boys in a popular bar/restaurant in West Hartford Center, not far from my house. We'd get together for a bite and a drink or two over some great conversation: everything from how season two of *Homeland* was shaping up, to what our kids were up to, to how they were stripping Lance of his Tour de France titles.

Two weeks in a row there, we said hello to the same group of acquaintances. Kristin was in that group: a young, beautiful woman with a kind face and an outgoing, cheery disposition. The second time we bumped into her, I asked her for her number. She gave it up, but didn't think I'd remember it—'cause I didn't write it down. But I had already committed it to memory. When I called her, I didn't feel a ton of enthusiasm flowing back at me.

For a while, we just talked on the phone. She agreed to meet me for coffee. We started seeing each other maybe once a week—what I call our "huggy phase." We'd part company with a hug each time. I really didn't think she was into me. I know now she was just being cautious with this older guy (I've got twenty years on her) whose intentions she wasn't sure about.

Gradually, she warmed up to me and we started dating. In some ways, we're opposites: She's an extrovert, and I'm introverted. But she does share my jones for working out—she could kill it in the gym.

After a few months, though, I started to feel not right. I couldn't pee. I'd feel like I had to go, but . . . nothing. *Uh-oh. Here we go again?* Back to the docs I went. I had to undergo something called a TURP procedure, where they put an instrument up your urethra to remove the part of the prostate that's blocking the urine flow. Guys, you know how you dread that prostate exam at your annual checkup? Well, I'll take ten of those in exchange for never having another catheter jammed up my manhood. When they tell you it's not that bad, only a little discomfort? Just say to 'em: "If it's so easy, why don't you have it done to *you* at the same time? C'mon, let's do it together!"

The first week in December 2012, Kristin and I went to New York together. My friend Barb took me to New York–Presbyterian for my follow-up appointment while Kristin, who worked for a Hartford insurance company, got work done at the hotel. That's when I learned that my old friend was back. There'd been a tumor on my prostate. I was going to have to start chemo again.

Once I got back home, I remember sitting in my darkened house—alone with the *Here we go again* news. This time, I wasn't shocked or numb. More . . . resigned. I didn't have a conscious moment when I declared this to myself, but I was aware that my confidence had taken a hit. This is what cancer does—its relentlessness bears down on you and shakes your self-assuredness. When I was first diagnosed, like a rookie in his first turn around the big leagues, I didn't know what I didn't know; I was confident that I could ultimately rid my body of these rotten cells. I was all *Game on*. But each setback chipped away at that. Now I had to admit to myself: This was my life. Unless a plane I was on went down, this was how I'd be going out. And it might be soon, certainly sooner than I'd ever imagined.

I couldn't putter around the condo all night. I called Kristin, who, unknown to me, had been crying all day on *her* sofa. We met in West Hartford Center, in my car. We just sat there. I wanted to play her some songs. That's not right: I played her some songs, but I wanted to play her *one* very specific song.

It's a song written and performed by my buddy Javier Colon, the winner of the first season of *The Voice*. It's called "Okay, Here's the Truth." It's about a husband who thinks his wife is cheating. So we sat there, Kristin and I, in a parked car on the street, both of us crying and listening.

> *Okay, here's the truth*
> *It's gonna sound kind of strange*
> *But I took a new way home from work for a change*
> *It started out fine*
> *Till I got to Route 9*
> *Went an hour the wrong way before I realized*
> *I'm sorry I ruined all our plans*

I was hoping that you'd understand
Standing there watching her secretly talking
It is just about all I can bear
Now I know why she's been wearing
More makeup and caring
So much about changing her hair
The telephone vibrates on the table again
Another damn private call coming through
And now she's visibly shaken
And I just feel like taking that phone
Throwing it clear across the room
She answers "hello"
A man's voice I don't know
Says "It's time that you tell him the truth"
Now I can't take this no more
Honey, I'm out the door
No, I won't relax
I've got my suitcase all packed
But what she said next stopped me dead in my tracks
Okay, here's the truth
It's not what you think
The man that you heard is head of oncology
I'm sorry I lied
To you all of those times
I didn't know how to tell you
I might not survive
Okay, here's the truth
I've got six months to live
I only wanted what's best for you and the kids

I promise I'll fight
With all of my might
But if I lose this battle
I lived a good life
So baby just please hold my hand
And tell me that you understand.

We sat there for hours. I think I played her the song to let her know what I was feeling—and to let her know what she was in for, if she wanted to stick around. This is the deal. This is it. It's constant. The hurt is constant, the worry is constant, the stank of it is constant.

I don't project when it comes to other people's behavior. So I didn't expect her to stay or expect her to run. I was ready for either. But I wanted to encourage her to run. Why? Because I love her and this is a load, man. You're not prepared for it—whoever you are. You're not ready for this. No one is ready for this.

"You must not have known me too well," Kristin, who had been a caregiver in her own family, would tell me later. Because bailing never crossed her mind. A few days later, I was supposed to start chemo. Again. Kristin was going to meet me at the infusion center. That morning, I called her.

"I'm not going," I said. I wasn't up to it. Not again. Screw this. This is why I hate it when people talk about bravery and courage. Man, there have been hundreds of times I quit. Or wanted to. This was one of them.

"Stuart," Kristin said, "I'm getting in my car now and I don't have the address. You'd better text me the address, otherwise I'll just be driving around Avon."

I told her she needn't come—I could go through this alone. "Sorry," she said, "that's not an option. You're not going alone. We're in this together now."

I wanted her to bail. Because I really didn't want her to start— and then quit. This wasn't a part-time thing. You can have a hundred people tell you what it's like to be a caregiver to somebody who has cancer and you still won't grasp it. It's bigger than you think.

She was signing on to have a relationship with a single dad of two girls, twenty years her senior, who has cancer. Them's some issues, right there. But Kristin's all heart. She may have more heart than sense. Whether she knew it or not, there were now three of us in this relationship: Me. Her. And cancer.

CHAPTER ELEVEN

TWO DATES AND A DASH

As 2013 moved on, Kristin spent more and more time at the condo. On days I didn't do MMA (and sometimes even when I did), we'd either do P90X together or I'd dig out my old *Rocky* sound track and put on the familiar soaring sounds of "Gonna Fly Now," and we'd both put on big leather gloves and spar right in the living room.

That's right, I had me a regular sparring partner now. I know I had a few pounds on her, but she's wiry and tough. And she's an athlete. Despite her sweet demeanor, she'd compete. She clocked me good a couple of times.

Soon, Kristin would take a leave from her insurance job and move in. That was a big decision for us. She was adamant: "I never want you to face any appointment, any surgery, any procedure alone," she said.

But taking a leave from her job was a huge step. It's what I needed, though. When you're sitting there in your oncologist's office, it's hard to wrap your head around what you're being told. But Kristin would be there with me—and she'd be taking notes. She became more of an expert on my treatment and meds than I was. I could have dived in, but it would have been overwhelming. It was a relief to just sit there and experience the emotion I was feeling as my doctor talked to me.

This is what caregivers do. They're the forgotten ones in the cancer fight. Let me tell you, they're there every step of the way, often for little or no thanks. They suffer, too—but people seldom think of the caregiver when their hearts go out to those battling cancer.

Relationships are hard enough when cancer *isn't* in the picture. When it is, it impacts things in big and small ways every day. For example, one thing it's taken me a while to learn is that having cancer means having to be selfish. Ever since my first round of chemo, I've had neuropathy, a numbing in the hands and feet. That means I'm always cold. So when Kristin's comfortable and I'm freezing, I've got to get comfortable and she's going to have to be hot—just one of the countless compromises she's made. If we're in the car, I'm freezing if it's 74 degrees. I need it to be 80 degrees—which means she's sweating.

On Sundays, Kristin visits her dad, and I'm sure she'd like to have her boyfriend with her. But I do *SportsCenter* on Sunday nights, and I know the best prep for me is to do nothing during the day. I'll get in a morning workout and then lie around until I'm Bristol-bound. I know that if I'm on my feet all day, I'll burn out by ten o'clock at night. And I know the difference between doing a sportscast rested and doing it tired: When I'm rested, I'm really good at what I do. When I'm tired, I slump in my chair and close my eyes on the *SportsCenter* set when we go to commercial and try to summon the adrenaline I'll need to take the show to the next level.

Man, sometimes I just want to be silent. I talk a lot at work, then I'm looking into the camera and talking, then I'm "talking" on Twitter. When I don't have to talk, guess what I like doing?

Just being silent. When you're in a relationship with someone, though, they want to talk. It took Kristin a while to realize it's not that I'm mad or in a bad mood—sometimes I just don't wanna talk. And when I do talk to her, I always want it to be an authentic conversation. I don't want to talk for talking's sake.

Probably the biggest reason I like just being silent is that what's on my mind is cancer. That's what's there. It doesn't leave. I can't make it leave. I can't act like it's not there. Some people say, "Put it out of your mind." Man, *you* try putting it out of your mind. That's a Pollyanna world. You don't put this out of your mind, not when you're peeing blood and your stomach is churning all the time and you always feel like this thing is *inside* you, moving, growing, taking over. I can fake it—but I ain't gonna fake it with the people I love.

Sometimes I'll start to tell Kristin something about my cancer—how, this one day, I couldn't stop thinking about that day when the *Lawd* comes to take me, and I started to worry: How complicated would the estate paperwork be for my girls? Would they be okay if that dragged on? . . . and then I'll just stop.

"Tell me about it," Kristin will say. Or: "You don't talk about it. You don't let me in."

'Cause I feel like a damned broken record: "I'm scared; I'm going to die; my stomach hurts." That's *every* day. Why would you want to hear that over and over again? Man, I'd rather just be quiet. I'd rather just play golf.

That's pretty heavy stuff to put up with, no? That's what I mean when I say there are three of us in this relationship. Just like cancer is always with me, it's always with Kristin. Yet she remains so positive about life. She likes to say that your life consists of two dates and a dash—so you'd better make the most of the dash.

So . . . we do. We travel all over; whether we're at the Ritz-Carlton Dorado Beach in Puerto Rico or kickin' it on the Spanish Steps in Rome, we're making the most of the dash. I know it may sound like I'm liking cancer—trust me, that's not the case—but it *is* one of the things the disease gives you: an awareness in the moment of what truly matters. Whether we're looking out at the waves hitting the shoreline in Laguna Beach or just sitting at home watching TV, I'll look at her and think: *These are the moments I love.* Before cancer, I would have fun—but I wouldn't stop and take note of the moment. This is especially true for our simple pleasures at home. We'll spar or do P90X and then lie on the floor for dinner and watch *The Walking Dead.* Nothing could be better for my spirit.

THE 2013 NBA FINALS were shaping up to be a series for the ages. Since 1994, when the Houston Rockets clamped down on the Knicks' John Starks, there had been only two Game Sevens: in 2005, when the Spurs outlasted the Pistons, and in 2010, when Kobe's Lakers handled the Celtics.

Now the Heat and Spurs would make it three, after LeBron pulled off an overtime Game Six win in Miami. The series was the first in twenty-six years that featured four former Finals MVPs (Duncan, Parker, Wade, and LeBron). And it was also a sign of the changing times: a record ten players on the two rosters were of international flavor—pretty cool. What wasn't cool was that I wouldn't be there for Games Six or Seven. I watched from a bed at New York–Presbyterian Hospital instead.

During the Finals, I started having stomach issues, a lot of churning and bloating. Before Game Five, on Father's Day, I had a full-on blockage. I was in severe abdominal pain. I did the pregame show and then spent the rest of the game lying down in the production trailer. I pulled it together enough to be able to do the postgame interviews after Danny Green went off from downtown to beat the Heat. It was two a.m. when I was done with work and I told my bosses: "I don't know if I'm going to make it to Miami."

I was in constant pain. It may have been due to the scar tissue that developed after the last two surgeries or it could have been another tumor—we'd never know if I didn't head back east. So I chartered a plane, and once we landed in New York, I went straight to the hospital.

The scans showed nothing. As Dr. Milsom explained, that didn't mean there wasn't a new tumor—just that he couldn't detect it. And he didn't want to open me up again unless he absolutely had to because that would only ultimately create more scar tissue—it was a vicious circle.

Instead, they treated me with meds and I watched the Finals in my room. That's when, after Game Seven, I watched my colleague Doris Burke host the trophy presentation. As I mentioned, she's a pro and she did well, but, damn it, that's my job.

By the end of summer, I was still having regular flare-ups. My stomach had hardened and you could see rises in it. I called Dr. Milsom: "I know you don't want to go in again—"

"No, it's time," he said.

This time, I was headed for the mother of all surgeries. It took ten hours. There was a cancerous tumor and a ton of scar tissue that came out. Afterward came the pain. I was in the hospital for sixteen days—every one of those nights, Kristin slept on a cot in my room.

I had an IV, some type of special IV, an epidural for pain, and other wires coming out of everywhere. The worst was waking up with a catheter in my manhood. Man, I'm telling you: If catheters are playing the Ku Klux Klan in a football game, I'm rooting for the Klan. I had to have three different catheters put in during those sixteen days. It was hellacious, the most crucifying, intense pain I've ever felt. I stuck a cloth in my mouth and screamed when they put it in. Then they take it out to see if you can pee on your own. I'd start to pee, but then the flow would cut off—so back in went the catheter. And, to top it all off, my old friend the Wound VAC was back—and would be with me this time for eight whole weeks.

My mom is a worrier. I had told her she didn't need to be there for the surgery. But Barb, God bless her, chartered a plane for my mom and dad to fly in, and she put them up at her house in New York City. Susan came in and gave the medical team hell when I was too weak to speak for myself.

But even with all this love around me, I had my moments of total despair. "I'm tired, I can't do this anymore," I'd tell Kristin. "It hurts too much." What an SOB cancer is. I'd now had three major surgeries in five years, not to mention a few minor operations and multiple chemotherapy treatments. It hit me: *This is what it's going to be forever.* I grew less confident about having many more years. Cancer is so relentless, you can't help but start to question your faith.

But, somehow, it's never a total loss. I had more of those moments of despair in the aftermath of this surgery, when I was down, crying, pissed . . . but then something would happen and I'd start to rebound, ever so slightly at first.

The girls would pick me up. When I used to do P90X in the living room, Sydni would roll her eyes. I'd monopolize the TV. "You're so weird," she'd say before going to her room. Now, when I was going home attached to the Wound VAC, back down to 160 pounds, she asked, "Dad, aren't you going to do P90X anymore?" It was like—no matter how annoyed she was before— she *needed* me to be that strong again.

It took a couple of months to get back. This was the hardest comeback yet. By Thanksgiving, I was supposed to be on a new chemo. But I wasn't ready. I felt so battered by my surgery, I didn't feel strong enough. As fall 2013 gave way to winter, I don't think there was a moment that I made the conscious decision not to do chemo. I just wasn't emotionally ready. I was still skinny and traumatized. I needed time to heal.

My doctors told me of two other options I could consider. One was a chemo drug called Erbitux. It's strong—the only concern was, would it be too strong? In a high percentage of cases, it causes disfiguring acne. In 2 percent of patients, heart attack or sudden death occurred after the first dose.

Some of my doctors recommended it. Dr. Baker was lukewarm on it. I couldn't get past the disfiguring acne. "You can always wear makeup to cover it up," Dr. Shah told me. "The people who love you, they're not going to mind."

I told him it's not about them—it's about me. It wasn't just that I'm on TV—though that's part of it. It's also that I know me. The doctors made it clear we're not talking about a bunch of pimples. The word they kept using was "scarring." Here's the thing: No doubt, makeup could cover up the scars when I'm on TV. But I know me. I won't go out of the house if I'm all messed up. I just won't. From the beginning, I pledged to do everything I could to beat cancer—but that I wasn't going to sacrifice my quality of life. I was still going to live my life. I knew that disfiguring acne would keep me from doing that.

They also told me about a clinical trial being done at Johns Hopkins in Baltimore. It's for a new type of medicine that has some promise, my doctors said. I applied and didn't get right in but hoped to be accepted in a few months.

Just after New Year's, I was starting to regain my strength when my friend, Nike's Amy Bartlett, called to pitch an idea. "If you'll let me," she said, "I'll round up a group of friends for a golfing trip to Florida. You don't have to be Stuart Scott. In fact, there'd be one rule: No one is allowed to talk about cancer." She said it would be like a grown-up Make-A-Wish weekend—golf and people I love.

I was resistant at first, but, man, I'm glad I went for it. We stayed at the Breakers Hotel and Resort in Palm Beach. Kristin and I were joined by Amy; my buddy Brian and his wife, Ericka; Doug Ulman; and our friends Michelle Bemis, who helps run Tiger's foundation, and Shannon McGauley. We played golf in the rain, giggling the whole time. "When it rains, you dance in the rain," Amy said.

Amy called Tiger and got us onto the exclusive course at nearby Medalist Golf Club. It was designed and founded by Greg Norman in 1995. It's probably appropriate to pause here for a word about my golf game: I have a picture-perfect swing. But the overall game? Not so picture-perfect. My short game is okay, but I can be a mess off the tee. Andrew Copeland of Sister Hazel once said when we were playing: "That's the prettiest swing I've ever seen on a crappy golfer."

Anyway, Tiger, Medalist's most famous member, lives about twenty minutes from the course, on Jupiter Island. When Amy told him we were in town, he met us at Medalist. We hung out and had some great laughs. He didn't play with us—probably afraid of being shown up by a cancer patient.

BACK HOME, I started an oral chemotherapy in March that tore me up, man. I'd gotten back up to 169 pounds, and then I started this oral treatment that had me running to the bathroom every half hour. I quickly dropped back down to 160. And I mean quickly; Kristin and I were getting ready to go to Hawaii—making those dashes between the dates worthwhile—and I got my clothes taken in before we went. Midway through our trip, we noticed that my pants were *already* loose in the waist.

I gave up on the chemo after a month. I'd wait for the clinical trial. I concentrated on getting my body back to a healthy state:

If my body felt good, the mind would follow. So back to my real medicine I went: a steady diet of MMA, P90X, and sparring.

Soon I was feeling like me again. I got back to 170 pounds and was starting to look cut again. I took a photo of me flexing and sent it to my mom, my dad, my sisters and brother, with this note: "48 years old. Cancer Survivor. Father. Son. Brother. Friend. I couldn't have got back here without you all and without you all showing me the love that you all have shown me. I just want you to know I'm still working and trying to beat this thing. Holla, Stuart."

Again: It's funny, what cancer gives you. It makes you more open emotionally, more vulnerable. Before I got cancer, I'd never have sent such an earnest note to my family. Oh, I would have taken the photo of me flexing, but I would have sent it to my brother, Stephen, just to give him a hard time. And the note would have read: "Yo, dude, come get some of this."

Because even though we were now both middle-aged men, Stephen and I still competed and talked trash. Once, when I was pretty cut and Stephen was all fat, I said, "Man, I didn't know you was pregnant." That got his butt back into the gym right quick. If we're in front of a mirror with each other, one of us will say, "Man, I'm bigger than you"; the other: "Damn, I'm more ripped than you." That's what we do.

As summer approached, everything seemed to happen all at once. The NBA Finals were once again approaching—it would be a rematch between the Heat and the Spurs, and a chance for me to make up for missing out on the last two games of last year's series.

I got accepted into the clinical trial at Johns Hopkins—so I'd soon start flying to Baltimore for an infusion every other Monday.

And, one day, Maura Mandt called to give me some news. Maura, executive producer of the ESPYs, is one of the most connected women in entertainment. She is also highly feared. She takes charge—if she were a man, everyone would be talking all about her leadership skills. But I also knew what few others did: that, somewhere behind that Type A personality and the barking orders, was a real soft spot. She was calling to tell me that, this year, I'd be the recipient of the Jimmy V Award for Perseverance at the ESPYs.

Man, I'd *presented* that award. Now I was going to get it. I was stunned and honored and even a little embarrassed: I didn't feel like I deserved it. I was just doing what I had no choice but to do.

But then I thought of all the cancer fighters I could represent that night, and I realized getting the ESPY didn't have to be about me. It could be about this army of fighters I've been in for the past seven years.

It was going to be one helluva summer.

CHAPTER TWELVE

POUNDING THE ROCK

S pend as much time as I have in professional sports team locker rooms and you're bound to see a whole lotta motivational quotes on the walls. They tend to be either part of the scenery or cringe-inducing clichés: Yeah, yeah, I get it, there's no "I" in "team."

But the San Antonio Spurs have this different kind of quote up in their practice facility, from Jacob Riis, a nineteenth-century journalist and photographer I'd never heard of: "When nothing seems to help, I go look at a stonecutter hammering away at his rock, perhaps a hundred times without as much as a crack showing in it. Yet at the hundred and first blow it will split in two, and I know it was not that blow that did it, but all that had gone before."

Now, that's deep. When they dismantled LeBron's Heat in the 2014 Finals after coming so close the year before, the Spurs were all about what Riis was talking about: They were resilient, relentless, prepared. Try as he might, LeBron couldn't rattle them; the Spurs were unflappable 'cause of all the rock pounding that had come before.

Like I said, I was pulling for the Spurs in that game, for personal reasons: so I could fly home with Sydni and do the clinical trial at Johns Hopkins. But after the Spurs took the title in Game

Five, and after the trophy presentation with Sydni just off-screen, I realized how much I admired this Spurs team. It wasn't about me, but I'd be lying if I didn't say that the moment was meaningful to me. A year ago, I had to watch this from a hospital bed. Now it was Father's Day, and my baby girl was with me while I did my job.

When Tim Duncan sat down with me for a postgame *Sports-Center* interview, he came with his two kids, Sydney and Draven. Sydni and I took a photo with them. Duncan has been called "the Daddest star of the NBA," and I could feel him on that. Just as I was celebrating with my girl, he was basking in the moment with his kids.

Not to overthink this, but back to that quote: We'd both fought back to get to this moment. But this is why I love Duncan and the Spurs: They ain't about the drama. When I asked Timmy what the difference was between this title and his first one back in 1999, he didn't get all theatrical about it. He simply said: "About fifteen years, I guess." That was funny, but it also felt familiar to me. Kristin teases me about how often, when talking about my medical situation, I'll say: "It is what it is." 'Cause that's the truest thing I can say. This is the deal. Gotta handle your business. Gotta keep pounding that rock, and maybe, one day, it will split in two.

MY FIRST CLINICAL TRIAL session was uneventful, but before my next one I developed another urinary blockage. So it was time for another look-see in my manhood. The morning we were supposed to leave for Rhode Island for Sydni's playoff soccer game, I had another of those *I can't keep doing this* moments. My urologist, Dr. Kennedy, knowing how I hate this stuff, had me take a Valium before the procedure, which consisted of a catheter-like microscope being stuck down there.

But it didn't stop me from hating this. I was crying and gritting my teeth and telling myself I'd had enough. But this is also the thing about cancer: You never know when a funny moment will suddenly break the tension. After numbing me, Dr. Kennedy said, "You're going to feel some pressure."

For some reason, I flashed back to some comedian I once heard talking about a visit to the proctologist. "You're going to feel some pressure," his doctor said. "Yeah, I feel it—in the roof of my mouth!" the patient said. Through my tears, I started to laugh. Especially when I thought of something else from the same monologue:

Doctor: "Look, I'm going to be checking for blood in your stool."

Patient: "Doc, you stick that thing up my butt and I can tell you right now, you're *going* to find blood in my stool."

So I was laughing and crying—the literal definition of having cancer, right?—at the same time that the microscope was in for about forty-five seconds. They've seen the blockage, Dr. Kennedy reported. It may be scar tissue—they don't know. But we'll have to do another TURP surgery—that procedure I had once before, where they go in through the urethra to remove whatever's blocking the urine flow. That would be the following Monday. For now, though, it was straight off to Rhode Island.

So here's the interesting, surreal thing about cancer. You go from that—from having a microscope squeezed down your manhood, from crying, from laughing—to playing in a touch football game on the beach a few hours later in Rhode Island, with Sydni and her teammates and about five of their dads. You go from being in the hospital, where that antiseptic smell fills the air, making you gag in the back of your throat, and you're peeing blood after they've done what they do . . . you go from all that to standing in the sunshine, holding a football, throwing a tight spiral to your daughter, and you wonder, even after seven years of this happening: *Is this really happening?*

So what could I do? I could play. Hell, yeah, I played. I quarterbacked our team. Her coach knew his girls needed time away from soccer to bond with their teammates. We had also done this the previous year during the state tournament, and in that game I threw Sydni two touchdown passes, and she ran a kickoff around the right side, turning on them jets, for a touchdown. Now, this year, we were down 2–0, and she came to me.

"Dad, what should I do?"

"Go out there, split right," I said. "When I say 'hike,' run as fast as you can. I'll get you the ball."

She ran a classic go route, I launched the ball, and she timed her leap perfectly, catching it in the corner of the end zone. Later, on fourth and one at our opponents' seven-yard line, I sidearmed her the game-winner. Before I had kids, I didn't think I'd ever love anything more than playing football. But throwing a touchdown pass to my daughter in my sport . . . man, it's emotional. I started the day crying, and now I choked up for an entirely different reason. 'Cause if you're an athlete and your kid is doing something athletic with you, I don't have the words to adequately express how amazing that is. Whenever I see Sydni turn on those afterburners, I always think back to the same thing, back to when she was born, back to when she was a baby, this little thing. This tiny little person had grown into this amazing athlete. My little girl . . . was doing *that*. I fill up, man.

Later, after dinner back at the hotel, Sydni invited her friends to watch a movie up in our room. Ordinarily, the idea of a bunch of people coming to my room at nine p.m. to watch a movie? Absolutely not. But her feeling good enough and comfortable enough to invite five girls to our room? I loved it. Kristin and I went to the fitness room. When we got back, six girls were in one twin bed watching some stupid movie where bugs were coming out of Bradley Cooper's eyes.

It had been a long day, but now I wasn't tired. I was giddy. My baby girl told her friends, "Come to my dad's room." There was no way I was going to say you can't do that. My day started with a god-awful medical procedure, with me saying *I can't do this anymore* . . . but apparently I could. I'd been down. Sydni brought me back up.

BEFORE DAWN the following Monday, I was in the passenger seat as Kristin was driving me to the hospital for the TURP procedure. I had a hoodie on, looking all gangsta, rocking out to Slick Rick's old-school "Children's Story," when I shot a quick video to send to the girls.

"Hey, what's up, Monday morning, five-fifteen," I said. "On my way to the hospital to have a little surgery. Not big surgery but a little surgery. But I wanted you to hear the music I was listening to. Yeah. Mmmm-hmmm. Yeah, are you up? All right. I love you. Bye."

Sydni responded later with a text: "That's an ungodly hour to be awake, but a good song."

Taelor called later. "Because of you I had a nightmare," she said.

"What do you mean?"

"I woke up at eight with a nightmare that someone was attacking my eyes," she said, teasing me. "I think 'cause you sent me that, I had that nightmare."

I'd always tried to shield the girls from my fear, always talking to them about being strong, always seeming confident. They did the same with me, an interesting dance. But I knew what Taelor's dream was really about. She didn't have to tell me she was afraid; we were too busy putting up strong fronts for each other.

Two days later, I was back in Baltimore for round two of the clinical trial. And that's when all hell broke loose. Toward the end of the infusion, my heart started racing and I was getting shooting pains in my groin and lower back. But then it settled down. The next day, I went into Manhattan to get my suit for the ESPYs—I'd be receiving the Jimmy V Perseverance Award in a week.

But that night I started feeling weird. I was peeing blood, though that wasn't surprising, having just had the TURP procedure. But I also was up every forty-five minutes to pee during the night. Then I started to get severe stomach cramps. I thought it was simply because I'd eaten a bagel while lying down—

something that had bothered me before. But it kept getting worse. By Saturday morning, I was doubled over in pain and could barely walk to the bathroom. I thought this must be a tumor pushing through some wall that had been keeping it at bay. You know where I went with this, mentally: "I'm going to die soon," I said to Kristin. It's not a big step to get to that place, because it felt like my suitcase had been packed for that ride for some time now. My doctors told me to get to the hospital.

There, the pain went from my stomach to my back. Tests and more tests followed. They told me there were no signs of cancer in my kidneys or liver, but that . . . my kidneys were failing. And something was messed up with the liver. The combination of the TURP with the clinical study had triggered some kind of blockage in my urethra.

I was on some powerful drugs, so it's all a blur to me. But it was a crash, man. Four surgeries over the next seven days. Wires and tubes coming out of every part of my body—and I mean *every* part of my body. They put stents in through my back to clear out the kidneys.

Once the kidneys were drained, I started to feel a little better. Still, we didn't know what caused this. My stomach pain may have been "referred pain," I was told. Maybe the TURP–clinical trial combination triggered the kidney failure and that sent a signal to my stomach. I'd never heard of "referred pain," but okay . . . now how do I turn down the referral?

A week later, I wanted to go home. I was supposed to fly to LA on Sunday and I needed a few days to get ready. All week, my doctors were telling me they'd get me to Los Angeles. But now I sensed they weren't so sure. They wanted me to spend at least another day in the hospital. Barb called me, and I could hear the concern in her voice.

"Do you think you should be going to LA?" she asked.

"No, not really," I said. "I don't think I should be going."

Then I paused. "But, it's bigger than me, Barb," I said. I didn't know how it was bigger than me, but I knew that this was something I needed to do. "I'll go, but I'll be smart about it."

I knew I'd be tired, but when I got home from the hospital on Friday night, I was alarmed by how wiped out I felt. I'd had more energy the three times I'd come home after having my stomach sliced open and parts of my insides removed.

But that shouldn't have come as a surprise. "In the span of eight days," my surgeon explained, "your body has been assaulted about six times. The TURP, the clinical study, the surgeries in the hospital."

Maura and the honchos at ESPN did what they do. They called and said, "We're flying you, your girlfriend, and daughter out"—on the Gulfstream G450, one of Disney's state-of-the-art corporate jets.

I'd have a bed and a big bathroom. Five-hour flight equals at least five visits to the toilet. But even with the Gulfstream, I wasn't sure I'd make it. Sunday morning, taking a shower, I didn't have the strength to bring my towel over my shoulder. I just sat on the toilet, feeling defeated, and said, "Kristin, I can't."

She dried me off and dressed me.

Taelor had decided not to come. I wanted her there, but her summer semester at Barnard had just started. Sydni was missing the second week of her a cappella camp. On Friday, when I got out of the hospital, her mom brought her to the condo, and Sydni was upset. "I know I've known about this, but is there any way I can come out to LA on Tuesday?" Sydni asked. "Is there any way, please? There's this song; I have a solo." She wasn't being crappy about it, which I appreciated, but I told her there wasn't.

"Can we come back early?" she asked.

No. We were going to fly from LA to Raleigh to see my folks, whom we hadn't seen in five months. On the plane, I slept a lot. In between naps, I watched the World Cup on a flat-screen TV with Kristin and Sydni. Like I said, the plane was off the charts.

I HAD ALREADY WRITTEN most of my speech and committed it to memory. Remember, I've presented on that stage before, so I knew that I'd have to memorize: The teleprompters are too far away for me to read.

I had a feeling that something magical was about to happen. The more I thought about the speech, the more I thought it was okay to feel ambivalent about being honored. That maybe the best thing I could do was to *use* that ambivalence—to see this as an opportunity to stand for something bigger than me. To represent for everyone in that army of fighters that had linked arms with me for years now.

Another reason I felt like this week was going to be about something bigger was that so many of my friends and loved ones were coming out. And I wanted the people I love to share this. It was too much for my mom and dad to travel across the country, nor could my favorite auntie and my cousins Anthony and

David make it. Fred, my best friend since high school, would also be absent. But everyone else in my life would be there. I didn't even know exactly what they'd be sharing, but I wanted them to share it.

Barb was flying in, as was Laura. Somehow, after all these years, the two female friends I'd known the longest had never met each other. How could that be? My buddies Scott and Brian were coming out. Amy and Deedee would be there. Susan, Stephen, and Synthia. Jackie Barry, who used to run the Jimmy V golf tournament when it was in Raleigh—a dear, dear friend. My agent and close friend Jackie Harris.

Oh, and Jack Bauer would be in the house. When Maura first asked me whom I wanted to introduce me, I joked, "Denzel."

"What about Michael Jordan?" she asked.

"That'd be cool," I said.

She asked and Michael wanted to do it, but he had a scheduling conflict. "Anyone else?" she asked.

"How about Kiefer?" I asked. *24* was my favorite TV show of all time. When the series first ended in 2010 (before its return last year), I had downloaded the final episode and watched it on an airplane. I remember getting all choked up when Jack escaped from the Russians and thanked Chloe for always being there for him. I don't think I was emotional because it was such a great episode; I was moved because this character had been a part of my life for nine years.

Later, my boy Scottie and I got pretty deep one night, talking about why I related so to Jack Bauer. "My favorite TV shows are *24*, *NYPD Blue*, and *Homeland*," I said. "So some of it is my dad and law enforcement. Another part of it is that I've always enjoyed shows where the lead male character is a flawed but good person. But my inner twelve-year-old likes Jack Bauer 'cause he's a badass who kicks ass and doesn't follow authority. He just wants to do the right thing even if it means stepping outside the lines."

Scottie thought for a moment. We had first met fifteen years ago on the golf course and struck an instant bond. He saw that I had my kids' initials on my golf balls—T & S. And I saw that he had "ASC" marked on his balls: his kids are Alexis, Spencer, and Cooper. *I'm going to like this dude*, we both thought of the other. Then, when I found out he was into martial arts, too . . . it was all over. Blood bros.

Now he was thinking through my Jack Bauer hero worship. "See, I think for me, and I might have thought for you, it was in those first episodes years ago, when his daughter gets abducted," he said. "That's when I was, like, I'm down with this guy. 'Cause then it's like we say in martial arts, 'Today is a glorious day to die.' He's going to win or die for his daughter. We can feel that, right?"

Man, that's deep—I hadn't thought of that. But, yes . . . I've spent my whole adult life protecting my daughters—even protecting them from this damned disease tearing me up inside. Of course a badass character that does the same on TV would strike a nerve.

When Maura texted "Kiefer said he'd be honored," I was silly with excitement. While I was in the hospital the week before coming to LA, Maura texted Kristin just to check in and see how we were doing.

"We're fine; we're at the hospital, watching *24*," she texted back.

"Text me a photo," Maura replied.

So Kristin got behind me and took a photo of me watching *24* and texted it to Maura, who forwarded it to Kiefer: "Look what he's doing!" She forwarded me his text back: "What's he doing? Is he crazy?"

Jack Bauer watching me watch Jack Bauer. Cool.

WITHIN MINUTES AFTER ARRIVING at our hotel and checking in, Hurricane Maura was on the case. "What do you need?" she asked, on her way over. She burst through the door, staffers in tow, barking orders. "Stock the fridge with Gatorade," she told them.

I'm telling you, Maura *runs* stuff. A natural leader.

She asked if I was up for a short walk. Just across the way sat the ESPN production trailer. She wanted to show us the five-minute video, narrated by Kiefer, which would be part of my introduction. We took our time and made it over there. A film crew had hung out with us during my first clinical trial session, shot footage of me doing MMA, and interviewed Kristin and Sydni. But I hadn't seen what they'd put together yet.

The piece blew me away. It showed me at the clinical trial, joking around with the nurse, in the gym, watching from the sidelines as Sydni scored a goal. They interviewed my friend Laura Okmin. "All the things he does, as his close friend, I want to say stop," she said. "Stop working out so hard; stop traveling so much; why are you doing so many *SportsCenters*? But it's what keeps him going."

"I hear from people every day: 'He's on TV and he's doing

what he loves,'" said my boy Doug Ulman, echoing something he's always tried to get me to wrap my head around—the effect I could have. "They take strength from the fact that he has not been paralyzed by his illness and that he's decided to live life on his own terms."

Then came Sydni. "When people ask me, 'Are you worried or are you scared?,' I've never really been worried," she said, choking up. "Because he's always had the most confidence: He's always told me he's going to get through it and that we're going to get through it together."

Here's the interesting thing about Sydni in the piece. She was saying these words that she only felt partly—because she was crying as she said them. So she was mirroring me. Because I've always been telling her, "Don't be scared." I've been showing confidence for her sake—all this stuff I don't feel all the time. I feel some of it, yes. But I've got to show her that toughness all the time.

So, huddled in that trailer, I started to cry, feeling like I was watching a mini me. She was talking brave, but the fact that she was crying let me know it was more complicated than that—just as it is for me. Just like me, she was scared.

As Sydni spoke, the first notes of Sam Smith's "Stay with Me" played under her words. Soon, the music rose to a climax.

> *Oh, won't you stay with me?*
> *'Cause you're all I need.*

Later, Sydni would tell me that *that* was the song she was supposed to sing solo in week two of a cappella camp. Man, this was some kind of sign. Note to self: Find a way for Sydni to get back home in time to sing that song.

But first, as the video ended, I stood up, tears streaming down my cheeks. Maura and her staff had the foresight to quietly leave the trailer. And I grabbed Kristin and I grabbed Sydni and I pulled them tight. All you could hear was Sam Smith's haunting notes and all our sniffles.

"This is why I needed you guys here," I said, clutching them. "This is why I needed you here."

CHAPTER THIRTEEN

YOU BEAT CANCER BY HOW YOU LIVE

don't know, Laura," I said. "I don't know if I'm up to it."

While I was in the hospital, drugged and with tubes coming out of every opening in my body, Laura had called with an idea she and Kristin had: a group dinner on Monday night of ESPYs week. At that point, the way I was feeling, I would have said no to anything.

"Trust me," she said. "This will be your favorite night."

"Laura, I don't know."

"Trust me," she said. "You're going to love it."

What could I do? She wouldn't take no for an answer. And I thank God for that, because she was right. Monday night was one of the best nights of my life.

We took a limo to a Venice Beach address Laura had provided. It was me, Kristin, Sydni, Susan, Synthia, Stephen, Scottie, Brian, Deedee, and Barb; we'd be meeting Laura, her boyfriend Mike, and a few of our other close friends. In the limo on the way over, we signed Scottie up on Twitter—but for weeks he still couldn't figure out how to post something or follow anyone.

Once we got there, we found a rusty metal door on an old brick wall that was covered by a mural. What the . . . ? Once you opened that door, though, it was like you entered a different dimension. Inside, the downstairs of the house—which belonged to friends of Laura and Mike—opened onto a breathtaking alfresco courtyard. There was a bar, a stage, catered Mexican food.

I didn't have a lot of energy to be walking around, but that was fine—it wasn't about me. It was about all these people who love me, and whom I love. Laura brought out another surprise— T-shirts for everyone. And not just any kind of T-shirt. Gray T-shirts that read "Fuck Cancer #stustrong" in black lettering.

Holla! When Laura pulled out the shirts, we all high-fived. A bunch of us put them on, and we took photos and posted them on Twitter. Over the next twenty-four hours, it started to blow up. Comments followed comments; most thought it was pretty cool. Some objected to the language.

We talked about that as soon as Laura started handing out the shirts. If someone said to me, "Hey, would you want your daughter wearing that?" I'd probably squirm a little. But you know what? It's bigger than that. It's not about that one bad word. It's about the anger and the power and the fury behind what cancer is. You gotta spell out the word to get all that across.

Leave it to my big bro Stephen to have the line of the night when we were debating whether to have it spelled out. "Anyone complains, just tell 'em they're right—cancer really *is* an offensive word."

When someone on Twitter complained about the word, Susan responded: "Understand, it's personal and a choice. Got mad love for your right to feel that way."

I thought that was so smart. I totally get why you'd be upset if your kid saw that word on someone's T-shirt. But, in this case, it's the right word, man. It says: *We're not standing for this. We're fighting back*. Besides, your kid ever watch HBO? All right, then. Trust me, he or she ain't no stranger to the F-bomb.

The next day, Laura said we should print up a lot of them and sell 'em online, with the proceeds going to cancer charities. Brilliant. She got right on it.

Meantime, dinner was a blast. Tony Ferrari, a young crooner with a touch of old soul, was the entertainment. He's this baby-faced kid who can hit the high notes—his soulful cover of Sinatra's "New York, New York" killed it.

As Tony was singing I started to feel a little chilly. Someone brought me a blanket as I sat on this big ol' comfortable sofa, with Kristin on one side and Sydni on the other. While Tony sang, I FaceTimed Taelor so we could all share the moment together. I kept looking around at all these friends and loved ones. *Lucky*, I kept thinking. *I'm so lucky.* It was one of the best experiences of my life: to be with these people, listening to this music, loving this moment.

I had asked Laura earlier, "Hey, can Sydni sing with Tony?" She said sure. So they did a duet of a Christina Aguilera song. I also asked if they could do "Stay with Me."

Man, they crushed it. My baby girl got up there and . . . I started bawling, watching her. She belted it out, so poised and self-assured. When she hit that last note, everyone erupted—applause, hoots, howls. "That's my daughter! I taught her everything she knows!" I yelled.

This song was now, like, my anthem. You know what? As much as I wanted to see my parents, I knew I didn't have the energy to go to North Carolina after all this. When Sydni plopped back down on the sofa next to me, I said: "If we leave here Thursday after the ESPYs and go straight back to Connecticut, can you still do the solo?"

"I don't know," she said. "They gave it to somebody else. I don't think that would be fair."

I texted the lady who runs the camp: "Listen, if Sydni is back Friday, can she sing?"

"We'd love to have Sydni" came the reply.

So it was settled. We'd go back so Sydni could sing "Stay with Me." By the way, when she did sing it, a few days later, I noticed her hugging a young man after her part of the solo. The overprotective dad in me was ready to get in this young buck's face, or at least give him the ol' stink-eye stare. But then I realized: *C'mon. It's the middle of the afternoon and they hugged out in the open—nothing shady here.* So I slinked away.

But that would be later. On this night, protecting Sydni from an innocent boy was the furthest thing from my mind. As Laura buzzed around, as Tony Ferrari crooned, as Scottie mingled with friends of mine he'd only ever heard about, I put my arm around my daughter and thanked God I could bring her back to sing "Stay with Me." 'Cause she was smiling. And it felt right. It was some kind of sign that this song came out of nowhere to play such a role in my life in the past twenty-four hours.

MEANTIME, MY EGO GOT bruised while in Los Angeles.

Stephen, Scottie, Brian, and I were waiting in front of the hotel for our car. Now, picture us. Brian is 5'8", but he's a marine. Stocky, cut. Stephen is 5'10", a big, strong guy. Scottie's lean and in shape, and carries himself with that New York swagger. Pass him on the street and you'd give him a wide berth. And then there's me—skinnier now, yes, but still athletically built.

And, outside of Stephen, all of us were experienced fighters. Minding our business in front of the hotel.

That's when a pudgy guy in his early twenties came up first to Scottie. "Hey, can I borrow one of your guys' phones?" he asked.

Scottie stared at him. "Look, I'm from New York," he said. "I don't carry my phone."

The dude looked at me. "You're not using my phone" was all I said.

The guy walked off. We laughed about Scottie's response: "I'm from New York." Seriously?

"I was trying to be polite," Scottie said. "I never met Stephen before. Didn't want to create a scene."

As we were chuckling, the valet approached. "Hey, guys, listen," he said. "If anybody asks to borrow your phone, don't do it—they run off with them."

Huh? *That* dude was going to race off with *my* phone?

Welcome to our Larry David moment. The four of us stood there, stewing. We didn't feel like we'd dodged a bullet; no, we were *insulted*—how dare this pudgy little dude think he could rip us off and outrun us?

"He wouldn't be able to take a step," Scottie said. "Even in Stuart's weakened state, he would have been annihilated."

Now we *wanted* to give him our phones. We looked around for the guy. Our car had come, but we left it idling while we looked—phones at the ready. No luck. We couldn't stop talking about it: *Really?* You're going to steal from the four of us?

It became the week's running joke: "Here—take my phone!" But don't think we didn't keep our eyes out for the phone bandit. Man, I wish I could run into him even to this day.

That got my adrenaline flowing. So we headed to the hotel gym—I'd just do a light workout. Get the blood flowing. Half hour on the elliptical, maybe some curls. When we were leaving, who walked in but Michael Sam and his boyfriend, Vito. Michael was getting the Arthur Ashe Courage Award for coming out before the NFL draft.

First, let me say: It *was* courageous. If you know anything about the locker room, especially at the pro level, coming out is nothing but brave. It's great that Michael's teammates at Missouri were tolerant and supportive, but an NFL locker room would present many more challenges. We chatted with Michael and Vito—they're great guys. I'm pulling for Michael to land with an NFL team. Then Brian got a bright idea; back into the gym we all went.

Brian invited Michael and Vito to play push-up poker with us. For years, we'd been playing this game Brian made up at his gym. It's regular poker with a twist: Before doing a push-up you draw from the deck, and whatever the number on that card is, that's how many push-ups you do. If you draw the color red, you have to do double the number on the card; if you get a jack, the person behind you has to do fifteen push-ups.

It can get to be a lot, man. Don't tell my docs I hit the floor to do this. But I'm a push-up freak. After a while, three of us hadn't folded. It was just me, Brian, and Vito, still pushing-up.

THERE ARE 7,100 SEATS in the Nokia Theatre, but it feels like more. I'd been on the stage before and knew how daunting and nerve-racking it could be for someone to stand up there, in front of a crowd of people like that. I've been in crowded auditoriums, but the look of this one when you're on the stage can be pretty intimidating. The audience seems to kinda swoop upward—if you're not careful, you can feel small before them.

Now, I like being nervous when I'm about to speak before a big crowd. It's like I always told Sydni and Taelor: What are nerves? Energy. You can control your own energy. So take it and use it. How? Keep this in mind: That whole big crowd out there? What are they getting ready to do? Listen to you. They're there to listen to you. So slow down, take your time. Be in charge.

During the show, Kiefer came out, said some kind words, and introduced the very moving set piece. When it was through and Kiefer called me up onstage, I kissed Susan, Sydni, and Kristin— in that order. The TV camera only caught me kissing Kristin as I stood up to go. If you watch the broadcast closely, you'll see me stand up and ever so slightly hold on to the seat back in front of me to steady myself. That wasn't nerves so much as physical weakness.

The sounds of Sam Smith's "Stay with Me" mixed with applause. As I stepped into the aisle, I was channeling the energy of the crowd. Channeling it into a force. Taking that self-conscious, inner *Oh, my God* voice and turning it into: *I got this.* As I approached the stage, I'd done it; I had a swagger, that clutch confidence.

Walking up on that stage, my eyes locked on Jack Bauer's. I'd met Kiefer once or twice before, but didn't really know him. We hugged, and I said into his ear, "Dude, really honored that you did this."

"I watched that video," he said. "And I'm so honored to be here."

He handed me the ESPY, and I stood at the mic. *Game on.*

"You know, tomorrow, all my boys are going to be like, 'Yo, man, I saw you at the ESPYs with Peyton Manning, Money Mayweather, and KD . . .'" I said. "I'm gonna be like, 'Yeah, whatever. Jack Bauer saved the world and he introduced me.'"

At that, I pulled the old Jay-Z gesture, flicking dirt off my shoulder. "*24* is my favorite TV show of all time, so, Kiefer Sutherland, thank you very much. I'm very honored."

The crowd applauded and Kiefer touched his right hand to his heart.

I talked about how I didn't really feel like I deserved to be on that stage, in the same company with all the inspiring figures who had come before me. "Although intellectually I get it," I said, "I'm a public figure, I have a public job, I'm battling cancer, hopefully I'm inspiring, but at my gut level, I didn't really think I belonged with those great people. But I listened to what Jimmy Valvano said twenty-one years ago, the most poignant seven words uttered in any speech anywhere: 'Don't give up, don't ever give up.' Those people didn't. Coach Valvano didn't. I now have a responsibility to never give up. I'm not special; I just listened to what the man said."

I went on to praise the Jimmy V Foundation, pointing out that its work had led directly to the clinical trial the video had just shown me undergoing. And then it came time for me to make a distinction I'd been thinking long and hard about.

"You heard me allude to it in the piece. I said, 'I'm not losing—I'm still here, I'm fighting. I'm not losing,'" I said. "But I gotta amend that. When you die, it does not mean that you lose to cancer. You beat cancer by how you live, why you live, and in the manner in which you live."

I had to pause while the crowd applauded. This line would blow up on Twitter and be quoted in all the stories about the speech. Only it wasn't exactly what I'd meant to say. Here's the way I had written it: "You beat cancer by how you live *while* you live." It wasn't like I made a conscious decision to replace "while" with "why," but even as I did, I grasped the reason for the change: Taelor and Sydni. They're why I live, why I fight. I believe in God; I think he works through people. He worked through me giving that speech. He gave me the wherewithal to say what I needed to say.

The last line of that quote—"And in the manner in which you live"—was also ad-libbed. I chuckled later, thinking about it. Because while it sounds good in terms of the speech's rhythm, it doesn't really add anything: "How you live" is the same as "the manner in which you live." Here I was feeling and sounding all profound—and I was being redundant.

Next, I directly addressed others in the fight. "So live," I said. "Live. Fight like hell. And when you get too tired to fight, then lay down and let somebody else fight for you." I thought of all the folks in my corner. That's what they do for me: They let me lay down. I singled out, without naming him, one of my ESPN bosses, Mark Gross: "I got these amazingly wonderful people at

ESPN," I said. "I got corporate executives, my bosses, this is true, who will text-message, 'Hey, I heard you had chemotherapy today. Want me to stop by on my way home from work, pick up something to eat, bring it to you?' Seriously? Who does that? Whose bosses do that? My bosses do that."

I'd debated with myself: Do I talk about all I'd gone through in the past week? It wasn't pretty. But I had to keep it real. "But even with all that, the fight is still much more difficult than I even realized," I said. "What you didn't see in the piece is what's gone on probably the last ten days. I just got out of the hospital this past Friday. Seven-day stay. Man, I crashed. I had liver complications. I had kidney failure. I had four surgeries in the span of seven days. I had tubes and wires running out of every part of my body, and, guys, when I say every part of my body, *every* part of my body. . . . As of Sunday, I didn't even know if I could make it here. I couldn't fight—"

The crowd applauded—points for just showing up.

"But doctors and nurses could," I said. "The people that I love, my friends and family, they could fight. My girlfriend, who slept on a very uncomfortable cot by my side every night, she could fight. The people that I love did last week what they always do: They visited, they talked to me, they listened to me, they sat in silence sometimes—they loved me."

Writing the speech, I'd originally meant to single out every one in my corner by name. Once I saw the video piece, though, I felt that wouldn't fit. Still, there were some people I needed to talk about, like Kristin and the girls. And my big sister.

"I called my big sister Susan a few days ago," I said. "Why? I needed to cry. It was that simple. I know that I can call her; I can call my other sister Synthia, my brother Stephen, my mom and dad, and I can just cry."

What did I tell Susan when I called her? I told her I was tired. That I just wanted to cry. I was tired of putting on a front for people; they'd ask, "How you doing?," and . . . it was just too much to go into it. That I'd started going into work late and heading straight for my office so I wouldn't have to talk to anyone until I was on the set. Because having to talk about my cancer just kept coming, in waves.

Susan did what she always does: She listened. Once, after my surgery in January 2011, she took me aside. "You don't have to go through this again if you don't want to," she told me. "All you'll have to do is say it. And we'll get the best hospice care for you."

In that and so many of our conversations, she had a way of saying something that just let me exhale. When she said that to me in 2011, I didn't consider hospice. But it was a great relief just knowing that if I ever did, I wouldn't be letting her down.

When I told her I wanted to cry, she said: "You should cry." And I did.

Speaking of crying, I was afraid I'd break down when it came to the end of the speech, where I'd close by talking about, and to, the girls. I'd practiced this part hard, trying to keep my emotions in check. "The best thing I have ever done, the best thing I will ever do, is be a dad to Taelor and Sydni," I said, to applause. "It's true. I can't ever give up, because I can't leave my daughters. Yes, sometimes I embarrass them. Sometimes they think I am a tyrant . . . Taelor and Sydni, I love you guys more than I will ever be able to express. You two are my heartbeat."

It sounds weird, but as I said it, I *felt* it. Standing on that stage, I *felt* them in my heartbeat.

"I am standing on this stage here tonight because of you. My oldest daughter, Taelor, I wanted her to be here, but college sophomore, second semester summer school starting this week, baby girl, I love you, but you go do that. My littlest angel is here, my fourteen-year-old. Sydni, come up here and give Dad a hug, because I need one."

She didn't know I was going to call her up. She'd taken her shoes off under her seat, and now, stunned, she couldn't find them. She walked out to the aisle barefoot. As she strode to the stage—all eyes on her—I said, "I want to say thank you, ESPN, thank you, ESPYs, thank all of you. Have a great rest of your night and have a great rest of your life." I had been planning on ending with "Have a good rest of the night" when one of the producers suggested "Have a great rest of your life," which I loved.

The crowd stood, applauding. By the time I'd finished speaking, Sydni was in front of me, the notes of—what else?—"Stay with Me" filled the air, and then my baby girl was in my arms . . . and we held on tight. "This is why I needed you here," I said in her ear, repeating my mantra from when we first watched the video together forty-eight hours earlier. Man, we hugged tight. I didn't want it to end.

We turned toward Kiefer; he shook Sydni's hand and I swear I thought: *Man, this is so cool. My daughter is meeting Jack Bauer.*

"Sydni, I have two daughters," Kiefer said.

"How old are they?" I asked, as the three of us walked off.

"Twenty-six and thirty-two," he said, still addressing Sydni.

"I saw you in that video, and watching you up here, it made me think about my daughters. So thank you very much."

Afterward, we took an extended family photo on the stage. The hugs continued late into the night. *So lucky*, I kept thinking. *I'm so lucky*. In the coming days, I'd realize I did what I'd wanted to do. I wanted to give those in the fight permission to not always be at their best. That was the one overriding theme of the speech. That was my purpose. You can try to be Superman, you can try to do heroic things, but you don't *have* to. You can just be.

It was only weeks later that I realized I was also talking to me. Giving myself permission. Because what was to come would test even my fighting spirit.

CHAPTER FOURTEEN

DAD, IS THIS *IT*?

t didn't seem that complicated at first. Three simple words: "You have cancer." Sure, it was jarring, scary, and even life-altering. But at first it seemed pretty straightforward: There's something wrong with you physically. You're sick. Deal with it.

I didn't know seven years ago about the mental burden cancer places on you. The way everything from that moment on would be divided into before and after, the way cancer would always be on my mind, even at the most seemingly innocent of moments. The way the disease hijacks not just your life, but also your very definition of yourself, because you're always calling into question your relationship to this invading army of cells. You're always asking, *Who am I? Am I what Twitter says, this Superman cancer fighter? Or am I a helpless cancer patient who can't summon the strength to do a set of push-ups?*

This is what cancer does. It shatters your self-confidence and makes you question everything—including who you are. They were three simple words back in November 2007—"You have cancer"—but maybe the most insightful thing that was said to me was the very first, the doctor's setup to the news: "Things just got more complicated."

He didn't know how accurate that was. What gets complicated is your own view of yourself. Three weeks after the adrenaline rush of the ESPYs, I found myself asking questions like *Who am I?*

The little voice inside my head, the one cancer is so expert at messing with, was telling me: *You're a fraud.* It was only three weeks since an ABC headline raved "Why ESPN Anchor Stuart Scott Refuses to Let Cancer Win" and the *Huffington Post* reported that I was "bound and determined to beat cancer."

For seven years, I'd embraced this idea of myself as a warrior. And I'd just given a speech that said, in effect, it's okay *not* to fight if you don't feel like it. Yet here I was, in the weeks following the ESPYs, not really taking my own advice. I was spending my days on a bed on the living-room floor of my condo—where I used to do P90X and spar!—and I'd become what I always said I wouldn't: just a cancer patient. I'd lie on that bed for hours. No energy. No will. And getting deeper and deeper into a funk because of it.

I'd bought into the warrior myth—even as I debunked it in the speech. And I was having a tough time navigating between the two ideas of myself: the never-give-up guy versus the scared cancer patient.

My days were spent driving a couple of hours to and from Yale–New Haven Hospital for radiation to shrink a new tumor in my prostate. I'd come back home and all I could do was lie down. Scottie came over one night, and I told him of the desolation I was feeling now, this sinking, hollowed-out depression.

"I take a walk around here, I'll do some squats, I'll do four sets of push-ups, some curls, and it wipes me out," I said. "I'll do that every other day. Well, I'm an every-day guy. Even with cancer, I'm an every-day guy. So why aren't I doing this every day? 'Cause I'm in pain like I've never been in pain. I'm not this warrior everybody talks about on Twitter. I don't feel that right now. I feel like a skinny guy who has to wear a sweater all the time. A guy who is always tired. That's how I feel."

Scottie gets it. We both know what it's like to be a fighter. We talk all the time about walking down the street with our daughters. We're constantly on the lookout for trouble, sizing up rooms, taking stock—in case something goes down. We instantly look guys up and down: *Here's how I'm gonna handle you if you start something.* Even if they're big guys—big dudes go down as quick as little dudes when up against someone who knows how to fight.

Only now I didn't feel like that skilled fighter. I felt like a fraud.

"You know, in moments of crisis, ordinary people do extraordinary things," Scottie said. "Because they perceive what they're doing as ordinary. Medically speaking, I don't know how many people could have made it to Los Angeles. That was extraordinary. But that's lost on you."

I thought about it. "Nah, man, something's changed," I said. "The last four or five days, I've told Kristin, I don't want to do this. Like, if this is the next month or however long, it hurts too much. I'd rather say my good-byes to Taelor and Sydni, and everybody can say their good-byes in their own way. What else can I say? I'm just tired of it. I'm tired of it. I guess I could say, *Hey, this hurts, but I'm going to get through it.* But I don't feel that right now. Maybe that's why I'm sad and feeling like a fraud, because I can't get there and I always used to be able to get there. The very thing I did was get there. When I'd leave chemotherapy, I'd be here working out, hitting pads, even though I was exhausted. I'd say it and my actions would do it."

Funny, now I was looking back nostalgically on times when I *had* cancer, as opposed to times *before* I had cancer. I remembered that, a few years ago, I did a Savage Race event on a Friday—three days after chemo. Savage Race is like Tough Mudder on steroids: In it, I ran a five-mile obstacle course through mud, over blockades, and under barbed wire, before finishing by swimming in ice-cold water.

Then there was the time I chartered a plane right after chemo and flew down to Nantucket for Daddy-Daughter Week; my siblings came down, and we all did P90X the next morning on the front yard of the house we'd rented. I was proud of that.

Was I now trying this on, seeing what it sounds like to not be what Twitter says I am—Mr. Warrior Guy? Ironic that that was my message in the ESPY speech: "When you're too tired to fight, lie down and let others fight for you." Little did I then know that I was really speaking to *this* me, the one three weeks into the future, who was in the depths of despair in his living room. I rewatched the speech a number of times because I needed to hear that it was okay to not be this ferocious cancer fighter all the time. It was okay to just be.

Scottie told me about this time he tiled a room—one hundred tiles. Ninety-nine were perfect. One tile was kinda scratchy. Human nature being what it is, all he could fixate on was the scratchy one. He lamented it, worked on it. "I came to think that was my only tile," he said. Finally, he took in the bigger picture: *Look what I just did. I tiled this whole room!*

The funny thing about cancer is that—just like in life—you're never just one thing. Warrior or victim. Sinner or saint. It's more complicated than that, man. On this night, I was feeling low. On another night, I might be raring to do P90X. Who knows? Intellectually, I know that both are okay, but the struggle to get to the point that you *feel* that . . . it's exhausting. "Just remember that this is a journey," Scottie said. "You're in a process."

THERE WERE A LOT of articles written about me after the ESPYs speech, but there was one that I read and reread and talked about with my friends, one that helped me work through the two drives within me—fighting versus just being—and the guilt attached to either option. Eliza Berman was an intern at *Slate* whose mother had died of cancer. She wrote a piece headlined "The Most Moving Thing About Stuart Scott's Speech at the ESPYs."

It rocked me, man. It was like the writer got inside my head and exposed my thoughts and feelings better than I ever could. "Cancer is a 'battle,'" she wrote. "People with cancer are 'fighters,' and if they don't die from the disease, they are 'survivors.' . . . The problem is one of language. We have a tendency to foist heroism upon people with cancer in a way that might, at first glance, seem generous and celebratory. But it can also be damaging. . . .

"Saddling people with cancer with Herculean expectations fails to acknowledge that it is absolutely normal to feel afraid, to feel like you can't go on, to *actually want to give up* . . . ," she wrote. "'I'm not special.' This was the first bit of debunking Scott offered. It reminded me of the bewilderment my mom expressed at being treated as some sort of superhuman saint. 'Wouldn't you get up every morning and take your meds and deal with the side effects?' she'd ask. 'Wouldn't anyone?'"

She got my message—and, for weeks, her take on it, her parroting back precisely what I'd meant, was just what *this* cancer patient needed to hear. "This guy who the video showed in the (literal) boxing ring, and on the sidelines of his daughter's soccer game—even this guy sometimes can't fight," Berman wrote. "The world needed to hear that. Scott's public ambivalence about the superhero cape he's been given was a gift to all those who don't always feel like superheroes."

She even somehow saw through the tough-guy façade I put on for the girls. "There was still plenty of battle talk," she wrote. "But I don't blame Scott for that. . . . He is a dad, by all appearances thinking of his daughters before himself. If his outward show of strength is an effort to help them feel less afraid, then I applaud him for it."

Whoa. I've been written about a lot. I've never paid a lot of attention to what people wrote or said. I like to say that what you think of me is none of my business. So it isn't often that a piece could affect me so deeply. But when I was down, I went over that writer's words and listened to my own at the ESPYs, and, gradually, on some days—*some*, because this was a working-through—I started to notice a change. On some days, there were no *should*s on my mind. I should work out. I should just crash. I should put on a brave face. No, every once in a while, it was okay to just take a deep breath and be present.

FRIENDS HELP, too, man. Scottie's visit lifted me up. While we were sitting around, my boy Fred called. I saw the caller ID.

"Hey, man, whatchu doing callin' me?" I said.

"Who is this? I must have the wrong number," Fred said.

In a week, we were all supposed to rendezvous near Hilton Head, South Carolina, for Daddy-Daughter Week. Only I didn't have the strength to make it—and I had to be in Connecticut for radiation every day. So Fred and his daughter, also Sydney, would be coming here.

"Hey, man," I said, "when you come here, you gonna be doing the grilling every night. Because, you know, I'm too tired. I have cancer." I faked a cough and a moan to help sell it.

"Oh, man," Fred said. "Playing the cancer card."

We chatted a few more minutes. "Okay, man, I don't want to talk to you no mo'," I said. "Love you."

"Love you, bro," Fred said.

We didn't talk about *anything*, not really. But, hanging up, my mood was better. I actually started to throw a couple of play sparring punches Kristin's way. "You should come by more often," she said to Scottie. "I haven't seen him like this in weeks."

That's the thing—my conversations with my guy friends run the gamut from sports to deep, life-and-death issues. Before Scottie came over, I mentioned to Kristin that he was stopping by because he and his wife were going away for the weekend.

"Where are they going?" she asked.

"I don't know where he's going," I said.

"You didn't ask?" She was looking at me like I was from another planet.

When he arrived, I shared this exchange with Scottie—and he knew right where I was going with it: the difference between guys and girls. "It never dawned on me to ask where you're going," I said. "I trust, subconsciously, that if I need to know, or you wanted to share, you'd have told me. And, don't take this the wrong way, but I don't care where you go—just be safe."

He laughed. "You didn't decide not to ask," he said. "It's omission versus commission. You didn't think to ask me until Kristin brought it to your attention."

"Because where you're going this weekend has no bearing on our relationship at this moment—and if it did, you'd tell me," I said. "But what has bearing is 'Hey, I'm going out of town, I want to stop by and see you before I go.'"

We go from nonsense like that to some real depth. Like stuff having to do with our kids. For me, ever since this last hospital stay, I've been worrying about how Sydni and Taelor are dealing with my cancer. Sometimes I get the sense that they're in denial and mask it with a ho-hum "Dad's sick" attitude. I know they care. I just worry about the wall they put up.

Last week, Taelor surprised me with a glimpse behind the wall. We were talking on the phone. She could tell I wasn't doing well.

"Dad," she said, "is this it? Like, is this *it*?"

Whoa. "I don't know," I said. "I hope not. But I don't know."

She paused. "Will you tell me when it's it?"

"Do you really want to know that?"

Without missing a beat: "Yes, I want to know," she said. "I will prepare myself."

"All right," I said. "If I know when I know, I'll tell you."

She'd had a teacher and two aunts die recently, so she'd been working through death lately. Good for her.

"Here's the thing," I said to Scottie now. "What if I don't want to do that?"

"I was just going to ask you that," he said.

"But since she asked me, it's not my call," I said. "I'll do it for her."

"That's right," Scottie said. "It may be emotionally tough for you. But she asked you so that's it, that's the answer. You have to honor her request."

Interesting. As the *Slate* writer noted, I'd spent a lot of time trying to shield Sydni and Taelor from my fears. No surprise I had two girls who kept theirs guarded, too. Now came Taelor's request. A crack in our façade.

CHAPTER FIFTEEN

BASKING IN THE GLOW OF THE NOW

Remember how I'd grow silent with Kristin and others, withdrawing into myself? Not because I was moody or mad or depressed—though, at any given moment, I could be any one of those things—but because I felt like a broken record. My voice droned on and on: *I have cancer. I'm scared. I'm going to die.*

I grew more and more tired of talking about the disease. Thank God that Kristin, who had once considered nursing school, had become an expert on my condition and my meds. 'Cause I stopped asking questions of my docs and I stopped giving friends the nitty-gritty details when they'd ask, "How you doing?" It wasn't because I was in denial. It was because I was sick and tired of being sick and tired. And I couldn't stand hearing my own voice reciting the same things over and over again. Listening to me telling people about my meds, about my weight loss, about how, when I pushed myself to do a few lightweight curls, it would deplete my body of what little energy I had and I'd crash in a heap on the bed on my living-room floor—it made me want to shout at myself: *Shut up!*

Well, when I started writing stuff down, I promised to keep it real, so I've gotta confess: I'm feeling that way now, with you. I've been filling up these pages with this cancer talk, and it's gotten to the point that I can't stand my own voice. I feel repetitive and pathetic and self-centered. So I'm going to try to skip the medical update, man. I apologize if you've gotten to this point and you need the lowdown on what happened next to me physically. Go somewhere else if you want to hear about how a cancer patient's body decays, about how it betrays you. When you've lived it, you realize that the body's breaking down is the least interesting part of this journey.

Suffice it to say that in September 2014, Dr. Kennedy said, "We've got to get you to the hospital. These are serious symptoms." Back to New York–Presbyterian I went. This time, I was there for seventy-five days—you read that right—with Kristin on a cot by my side the whole time. Every time I thought I'd be going home, something would happen: blood clots, grotesque swelling in my legs and feet. I lost track of how many surgeries and procedures I had. At one point, I was in the intensive care unit to have two stents surgically implanted to keep my veins and arteries open. Had we waited another day for that surgery, I likely wouldn't have made it. (See? Try as I might, cancer still finds its way into our conversation . . .)

I went home two days before Thanksgiving, one day before all my siblings arrived in Connecticut to celebrate turkey and football. No one said it out loud, but the truth of the matter was it could be my last one.

You'd think seventy-five days in the hospital would be awful. And it wasn't fun. But there were many times I was grateful to be there. For years, I'd been racing against time, hoping to make it long enough to be there for my girls' aha moment when it came to our relationship and our lives together. Well, I'd made it, man.

THERE WAS NO MORE HIDING. I'd long struggled with the balance between protecting Taelor and Sydni from what I was going through and being honest with them about what I was feeling. Until now, I'd always talked about "beating" this thing—there's that battle-metaphor language again. And they bought into the whole warrior thing. After all, after each major surgery, when I'd come home looking all gaunt and tired, they'd see me get back in the gym and start looking like me again—putting on some pounds, getting some muscle definition, recharging. Full disclosure: I might not make that kind of a comeback now. I still didn't want to scare them, but I knew I had to level with them. "This is as serious as it's been," I told the girls during that long hospital stay. "I'm more worried now than I've ever been about my own mortality."

The first time they both came to visit me at New York–Presbyterian, their mom drove Sydni into the city and they picked up Taelor at Barnard, not far from the hospital. Taelor came bouncing into my room first, smiling. Behind her, I saw Sydni, my ex-wife Kim's arm around her shoulder, ever so slowly walking in, her face drawn and frozen in fear. You know how Scottie and I would bond over our instincts to instantly size up threats when we've been out with our daughters? We'd compare notes on how, in a nanosecond, we'd scan a room to take the measure of who or what might pose a danger to them, silently drawing up a worst-case-scenario game plan. Well, that instinct kicked in when Sydni was so tentatively shuffling into my room. I could imagine what I must have looked like to her: very thin, lying in a hospital bed, tubes and IVs coming out of every part of my body . . . I quickly jumped up and sat on the edge of the bed.

"Syd, come here," I said, patting the spot next to me.

She didn't look at me, but she shyly stepped over and sat down. I put my arm around her. She was shaking.

"Are you scared?" I asked.

She nodded yes. Her eyes started to brim with tears.

"I know," I said, softly. "I'm scared, too."

I squeezed her shoulder, and she leaned into me, ever so slightly. I don't have to tell you if you're a parent: It's the worst feeling in the world to feel unable to protect your child from hurt and fear. You want to make it all better, but you can't. All you can do is let her know she's not alone, that you feel the same way. And I *was* filled with fear—but also anger. This was why I hated cancer. Because it messed with my girls and I was powerless to stop it.

I started keeping them up to date on what the doctors were telling me. Before I had the stent surgery, I gave them the background. "We've been waiting on these stents from Europe," I told them. "They've never been used in the States before. *I'm* the clinical trial here. Mine will be the only intestine in North America with these stents in it. Hopefully, it'll open the blockages I've been having."

That was new for us—I was letting the girls in on the details of my care. I still tried to avoid scaring them, but I wanted to be open with them. No more bravado, false or otherwise. A lot of times, what I had to say was hard for them to hear. "You can see, I'm getting worse," I told them both individually.

As for the future, I could make no promises. "I don't know when I'm getting out of here, girls," I told them. "The doctors can't tell me. I still have blockages and swelling. I'd be lying if I didn't say I was worried."

They were scared, too, though they put a brave face on it. Once, when Kim came to pick them up, she texted me that she was waiting for them in front of the hospital. "How are they doing?" she asked.

"They're good," I texted back. "We had fun."

"You said they were good," she later texted. "Once they got in the car, they were in puddles."

Hmmm. "They were cool when they left," I texted back. "I'm in puddles every time they walk out the door."

I guess we were still protecting one another. But at least now I'd made them a part of my care. This wasn't just something happening to me—it was happening to them, too. And I was no longer shutting them out with false optimism.

We started to have these moments in that hospital room—real moments, emotional moments, silly moments. They'd come by, and Kristin would sneak off to Barb's apartment for a few hours so the girls and I could spend time together. In my whole life, I've never basked in the glow of the now more than during those visits. We could be watching some silly video on Sydni's laptop and I'd say to myself: *My girls are here with me now.* Taelor could have her head buried in a book: *My girls are here with me now.* Even when they started snapping at each other, I'd have a bemused smile on my face: *My girls are here with me now.*

Once Taelor went away to college in August 2013, I didn't see all that much of her. Oh, we'd talk, of course, but we were leading separate lives. That isn't a complaint—it's as it should be. When I was in the hospital in September 2013 for those hellacious sixteen days, I saw her twice.

But now something was different. She'd call and ask how I was doing. I'd tell her not so good. "I'm so sorry, Dad," she'd say. At first, she'd text and ask if she could come by. Then she'd just start dropping in. One night she came in all dressed up, holding two big bags. She'd been shopping and was meeting a friend to take in a Broadway play: Could she leave her bags here? Uh, yeah. It started to feel like, instead of a hospital room, I had a little condo and she had a key and she'd pop in whenever the mood struck her.

One time, we were hanging late at night and she started dozing off. I told her to lie down. "Dad, I'm not going to lie down in your hospital bed," she said. I coaxed her into it. She fell asleep, my firstborn cuddled up with me. I couldn't take my eyes off her—just like I did all those years ago, when I'd sneak into her room and watch her sleep.

Another time, she pulled up a chair by my bedside and opened a book. It was written by one of her favorite authors, Roald Dahl. "What are you doing?" I asked.

"You read to me when I was little," she said. "Now I'm going to read to you." I closed my eyes and her voice washed over me.

Just before Thanksgiving, I got word that I'd be going home. I could tell Taelor was sad. She was more withdrawn, her eyes downcast. She had a confession to make. "In a way, I've *liked* you being in the hospital," she said, sheepishly. "I can come see you a lot."

She paused. I thought: *I hate cancer, but it's given me gifts like this very moment.* "You're not busy like you usually are," my little girl said, her voice breaking just a little. "I can have you all to myself."

IT'S HARD TO PINPOINT the moment you hate cancer the most. There are so many finalists in that game. But there was one time during my seventy-five-day hospital stay that just might qualify.

Sydni was starting at a new school and she was making her varsity soccer debut. And I wasn't going to be there for it. "Dad, it's no big deal," she said. "We're not very good. We're probably going to get killed."

I said all the right "Dad" things about how important it is not to have a negative attitude like that, but the truth is I was feeling pretty negative myself. I lay in that hospital bed and wallowed. Cancer was keeping me from being there for my daughter. Pure hate.

But then something happened. My buddy Brian went to the game and FaceTimed me from it. Suddenly, I *was* there. I saw my little girl start at left wing. I saw her lead a rush in the first two minutes and push the ball wide of the net. I saw her barely miss a header in the first five minutes. *She's faster than these girls.*

A few minutes later, she juked her defender on the wing and kicked a ball low to the outside corner, beating the goalie.

"*SCORE!*" I yelled, at the top of my lungs—nurses and doctors raced in while Kristin and I screamed and high-fived and hugged. "My daughter scored a goal!" I said. Some of the nurses stayed to watch.

At halftime, with the score tied 1–1, Brian went to his car to charge his phone. I knew his kids had games, too: "Dude, this is a great present," I said. "But I don't want you missing your games."

"Don't be silly," he said. "This is fun."

Early in the second half, Sydni led a rush on the opposing goalie. She dropped a trailing pass to a teammate, who missed the shot. That's when I noticed it. *They're double-teaming her.*

Didn't matter, though. Five minutes later, another rush; Sydni banged it in. Now it was a party. Nurses were hootin' and hollerin' and high-fivin'. With six minutes left and her team ahead 2–1, Sydni led another charge. Can you believe this? A freakin' hat trick. My little girl was dominating. She was the straw stirring that drink!

To watch your girl, a freshman, dominate in a game of seniors and juniors on both teams is one thing. To watch her get taken out with two minutes left and see her swarmed by her new teammates, to see her accepted in her new school, that was another altogether. And to have seen it at all, despite cancer's best intentions . . . that's priceless, man.

Kristin put a hat on my head and took video of me to send to Sydni: "I'm so proud of you," I said. "The way you played, the way you hustled. Thank you for giving me one of the best days I've ever had at a hospital." And then I tossed the hat to celebrate the hat trick.

"Thanks, Padre," came Sydni's quick reply.

I started the day hating cancer with a passion, and I ended it with love bursting outta me. That's what cancer does: It messes with you, but it also makes your love so much bigger.

Speaking of big love: That hospital time gave me time with the girls, and it gave me time with God. It was an opportunity to practice my faith. I spent a lot of time praying, talking to Him. *You know what my will is. Give me the strength to accept your will. If yours is different from mine, help me accept your will. And, please, as much as you can, take care of Taelor and Sydni . . .*

Yeah, despite it all, despite the surgeries, the chemotherapies, and the pain, as I lay in that hospital bed after Sydni's stirring soccer performance . . . I felt *lucky* once again. How lucky was I? Lucky to have a girlfriend who loved me enough to sleep on a cot and watch an entire game on FaceTime; lucky enough to have an elder daughter who would come and read to me in my hospital room; lucky enough to have a younger daughter who faced her fears with me and showed courage and class on the soc-cer field; lucky enough to have a friend like Brian, to whom I texted: "I don't know how to say thank you. I love you. This was the greatest gift of my life."

At the time, I thought: *Cancer tried to keep me from seeing Sydni's game, but I won.* But if there's one thing I've learned from this journey, it's that it's more complicated than that. To paraphrase a suave-looking dude you all saw at the ESPYs, you don't beat cancer just by living—you beat it by *how* you live.

Call me a sap, but I love to watch old couples, walking hand in hand or arm in arm. Eating at a restaurant and actually *talking* to each other. The wife leaning her head on her husband's shoulder. I see that and it assures me there *is* something as real as undying love. You know these people have gone through tough times, vicious arguments, sorrows, bad medical news, and yet . . . they've persevered. They got the *how you live* part.

I know now that I won't have the gift of many years, but I hope Taelor and Sydni conclude that that's the only thing I lacked. I know they will be kind and successful adults; that's been a given for years now. But I want them to take something else with them. I want them to take note of every moment and to make them count, just like those old couples that make me so sentimental. To refuse to live life on autopilot.

You know that saying I love? That life consists of two dates with a dash in between? I hope my baby girls take this with them: *Make the dash count.*

EPILOGUE

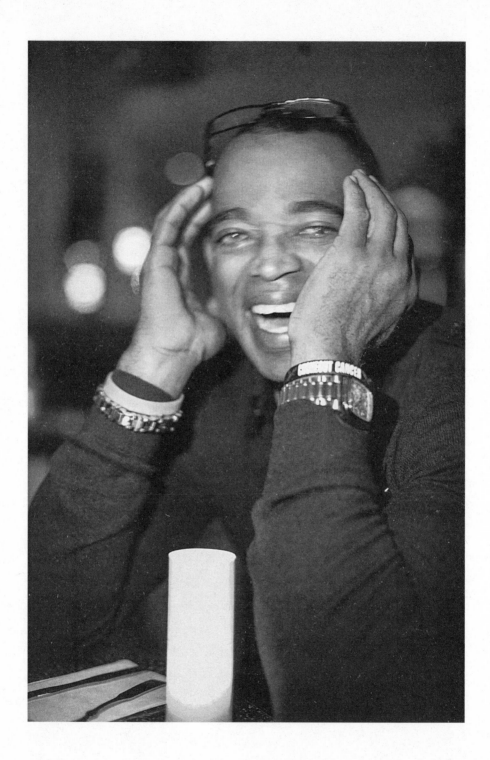

Stuart Scott spent Christmas 2014 with his daughters, girlfriend, and family. He delighted in every moment with his loved ones and never stopped plotting his return to television. Early on the morning of January 4, he passed away. Hundreds attended the funeral at Providence Baptist Church in Raleigh, North Carolina. As the casket was carried from the church, the sounds of the old-school song "Rapper's Delight" by the Sugarhill Gang filled the air.

ACKNOWLEDGMENTS

Everyday I Fight was a labor of love, performed by an all-star cast.

THE PROFESSIONALS

David Black is much more than the Michael Jordan of literary agents. For this project he served as Stuart's true advocate and visionary. The Black Agency's Sarah Smith was a consummate, ever professional problem-solver.

David Rosenthal's editing was rivaled only by his compassion and wisdom throughout this process. Stuart often described him as a "true mensch." His Blue Rider Press team often went above and beyond: production editor Janice Kurzius, art director Jason Booher, designer Claire Vaccaro, managing editor Meredith Dros, associate publisher Aileen Boyle, and editorial assistant Katie Zaborsky. I also want to thank Hannah Keyser for her invaluable research and transcription assistance.

The Personal

Foremost in Stuart's heart, Sydni and Taelor, his parents, Stuart's closest friends in the "Tribe," and his siblings, Synthia and Stephen, contributed tidbits, nuances, tone, and veracity in his absence.

Specifically, three special women contributed to finalizing matters in Stuart's absence. Kristin Spodobalski shared insights and support for many experiences chronicled in Stuart's last year. Under very trying circumstances, Susan Scott and Jackie Harris shepherded this project to completion, with great love, honoring Stuart and the way in which he lived at every step along the way.

Finally, a note about Stuart's lasting legacy: As the preceding pages illustrate, Stuart was about family and was aware of how privileged he was in his fight against cancer. When he fought and worked out he always believed he was fighting for himself and other cancer fighters. Stuart's wish was to continue the fight by starting a patient and family services foundation that gives cancer fighters and their families opportunities to lead normal lives—as he did throughout his battle. The Stuart "SOS" Scott Foundation, supporting cancer patients and families, will launch this year.

PHOTO CREDITS

INDEX

An index for this book can be found at
Penguin.com/EveryDayIFightIndex.com.

ABOUT THE AUTHORS

STUART SCOTT's groundbreaking style made him one of television's most influential broadcasters. As an anchor and commentator for *SportsCenter*, he became the face of ESPN, the most popular and recognized anchor of his generation. As lead host of the NBA on ESPN and ABC, as well as a host of *Monday Night Football* on ESPN, Scott redefined the telecasting of modern sports events. He received the Jimmy V Award for Perseverance at the 2014 ESPY ceremony. Stuart Scott died in January 2015.

LARRY PLATT is the former editor of Philadelphia magazine and the Philadelphia Daily News. He is the author of Only the Strong Survive: The Odyssey of Allen Iverson and coauthor of Just Tell Me I Can't: How Jamie Moyer Defied the Radar Gun and Defeated Time. His writing has appeared in GQ, New York, The New York Times Magazine, and Sports Illustrated, among other publications. He lives outside Philadelphia with his wife, Bet. You can visit Platt's website at LarryPlatt.net.